CW00617870

New Library of Pastoral Care
GENERAL EDITOR: DEREK BLOWS

Derek Blows is the Director of the Westminster Pastoral
Foundation and a psychotherapist at University College
Hospital. He is also an honorary canon of Southwark
Cathedral.

Going Somewhere

Titles in this series include:

New Library of Pastoral Care
GENERAL EDITOR: DEREK BLOWS

———

GOING SOMEWHERE

People with Mental Handicaps
and their Pastoral Care

———

Sheila Hollins
and
Margaret Grimer

First published in Great Britain 1988
SPCK
Holy Trinity Church
Marylebone Road
London NW1 4DU

Acknowledgements

The extracts from *Man and Woman He Made Them* by Jean Vanier,
published and copyright 1985 by Darton, Longman and Todd, are used by
permission of the publisher.

The extract from *They Keep Going Away* by Maureen Oswin is reproduced by
kind permission of the publisher, King's Fund Publishing Office.

British Library Cataloguing in Publication Data

Hollins, Sheila
    Going somewhere : people with mental
    handicaps and their pastoral care. —
    (New library of pastoral care).
    1.   Church work with the mentally ill
    2.   Pastoral medicine — Great Britain
    I.   Title   II. Grimer, Margaret   III. Series
    259'.4   BV4461

    ISBN 0-281-04336-1

Filmset by Pioneer
Printed in Great Britain by
the Anchor Press, Tiptree

*To all those people with learning difficulties
and their families and friends
who have shared their lives with us.*

Contents

Foreword

The *New Library of Pastoral Care* has been planned to meet the needs of those people concerned with pastoral care, whether clergy or lay, who seek to improve their knowledge and skills in this field. Equally, it is hoped that it may prove useful to those secular helpers who may wish to understand the role of the pastor.

Pastoral care in every age has drawn from contemporary secular knowledge to inform its understanding of man and his various needs and of the ways in which these needs might be met. Today it is perhaps the secular helping professions of social work, counselling and psychotherapy, and community development which have particular contributions to make to the pastor in his work. Such knowledge does not stand still, and a pastor would have a struggle to keep up with the endless tide of new developments which pour out from these and other disciplines, and to sort out which ideas and practices might be relevant to his particular pastoral needs. Among present-day ideas, for instance, of particular value might be an understanding of the social context of the pastoral task, the dynamics of the helping relationship, the attitudes and skills as well as factual knowledge which might make for effective pastoral intervention and, perhaps most significant of all, the study of particular cases, whether through verbatim reports of interviews or general case presentation. The discovery of ways of learning from what one is doing is becoming increasingly important.

There is always a danger that a pastor who drinks deeply at the well of a secular discipline may lose his grasp of his own pastoral identity and become 'just another' social worker or counsellor. It in no way detracts from the value of these professions to assert that the role and task of the pastor are quite unique among the helping professions and deserve to be clarified and strengthened rather than weakened. The theological commitment of the pastor and the appropriate use of his role will be a recurrent theme of the series. At the same time the pastor cannot afford to work in a vacuum. He needs to be able to communicate and co-operate with those helpers in other disciplines whose work may overlap, without loss of his own unique role. This in turn will mean being able to communicate with them through some understanding of their concepts and language.

Finally, there is a rich variety of styles and approaches in pastoral work within the various religious traditions. No attempt will be made to secure a uniform approach. The Library will contain the variety, and even perhaps occasional eccentricity, which such a title suggests. Some books will be more specifically theological and others more concerned with particular areas of need or practice. It is hoped that all of them will have a usefulness that will reach right across the boundaries of religious denomination.

DEREK BLOWS
Series Editor

Acknowledgements

In April 1986 a Day Conference on Pastoral Care was held at St George's Hospital Medical School. The speakers were:

Chris and Jo Dobson
Mary Jago
Professor Joan Bicknell
Professor Ron Taylor
Father David Wilson
Sister Stephanie Clifford
Dr Peter Helms
Rev. Lesley Turner
Alison Hutchinson
Rev. Ian Ainsworth-Smith
Dr Therese Vanier

We have taken last April's glimpse of how pastoral care might be offered and have extended it into the present book. The speakers are often quoted and we thank them for their vision.

Our text has been tested with the touchstone of experience and we are grateful for helpful advice from Therese Vanier, Ian McFarlane, Peter Gilbert and Rosemary McCloskey. Derek Blows encouraged us and proved to be an editor of initiative.

The Executive Committee of the Catholic Marriage Advisory Council granted Margaret Grimer a year to research the most appropriate ways for CMAC to offer pastoral care to people with mental handicaps, their families and their carers. She thanks them for their foresight and their trust in her. For Sheila Hollins, Professor Joan Bicknell is an unfailing source of support and inspiration.

Both of us are busy people and we recognize with gratitude that our book would have been much more difficult to complete without the patient and generous secretarial assistance of Freda Macey and Barbara Preston.

SHEILA HOLLINS
MARGARET GRIMER

One of Your People

Today people with mental handicaps are suddenly becoming more visible. All over the country and almost overnight it seems that long-established hospitals are being dismantled and sold. All over the country and almost overnight people with mental handicaps are to be found living in twos and threes and fours in ordinary houses in ordinary streets.

The more vocal among them tell us that they do not like our labels. Why should we keep referring to their handicaps? They are people first. They don't really like the word 'mental'. If we have to talk about their individual or collective needs why not call them 'people with learning difficulties'. The societies campaigning for them suddenly seem to be more aggressive: 'His greatest handicap could be your attitude'.

Men and women who exercise pastoral care within the community are beginning to ask themselves if they have any responsibility towards these newcomers. The director of a pastoral centre for people with mental handicaps is frequently telephoned by distant parish clergy: 'I have one of your people in my parish and I need your help.' His first reply is: 'Not one of my people. One of yours.'

This book is written for workers with any kind of pastoral responsibility (such people as clergy, teachers, social workers, hospital staff or counsellors) whose speciality is other than what is called mental handicap or learning difficulty. Part of the stock in trade of such workers is their inter-personal skills. Often they are good at listening, at responding with empathy, at offering understanding, counsel and comfort, at helping clients to examine options and to make informed decisions.

Most workers discharge their pastoral responsibility in a

highly verbal way. Their professional expertise may be to hold church services or to teach mathematics or to perform surgical operations, but when they are exercising a pastoral role they usually fall back upon the talking treatment. No wonder that they feel deskilled when confronted by a person with severe learning difficulties, with perhaps little or no speech, without facility in reasoning or in understanding cause and effect. No wonder that pastoral workers tend to think that such people belong to the speciality of mental handicap and are not really the concern of workers like themselves.

Yet in our time people with severe learning difficulties, supported by their parents, teachers and carers, are claiming their right to an ordinary life within the community. It follows that they are part of the clientele of each parish, each school and each hospital. They are present in each social services patch. They are as entitled as others to receive help when appropriate from counselling and charitable agencies, and not to be excluded merely on the grounds of their learning difficulties.

This can leave pastoral workers whose speciality is other than mental handicap in some difficulty. Much as they may wish to avoid discrimination, they can feel that at the very least they need some kind of specialized orientation before undertaking to work with people with mental handicaps. They need a sense of where they might be going.

When such pastoral workers do respond to the challenge of people with learning difficulties living in their midst they can meet further problems. Often they can feel isolated from their colleagues, who tend to praise their 'wonderful work' but show little desire to share it. They may also feel isolated from the experts, from those academics and teachers, those doctors, nurses and social workers who each at their own level have made a special study of people with learning difficulties. Sometimes a person who has a mental handicap will confront the pastoral worker with problematic sexual behaviour. Sometimes the pastoral worker's counsel is sought about ethical decisions concerning sterilizing a young woman or aborting an unborn child or giving minimal care to a newborn baby: does the fact of mental handicap change the guidelines completely? It is easy for pastoral workers who become involved with people who have learning disabilities to lose their usual sureness of touch and to be puzzled how to proceed or to fear that they may be acting inopportunely for lack of specialist knowledge and training. They need to know that they are going somewhere sensible.

This book speaks to both groups of pastoral workers, to those who have taken up the challenge and those who have yet to do so. It offers the orientation that they need. What is it like to have a mental handicap? What prospects are there? What about sexual behaviour? Is marriage a possibility? What can the churches offer? Is community care really possible? This book tackles all of these questions. It declares that people with learning disabilities are indeed going somewhere worthwhile, and it invites pastoral workers to share that journey.

In April 1986 the Section of the Psychiatry of Mental Handicap at St George's Hospital Medical School in London held its Annual Conference on the theme of Pastoral Care for People with Mental Handicap. The organizers had recognized that pastoral workers both within health care professions and from other walks of life were asking how the pastoral needs of people with learning disabilities could be met. The conference was attended by one hundred people including parents, social and community workers, clergy, lay parish workers, residential care staff, a marriage guidance counsellor, psychiatrists, psychologists, teachers, nurses and a few doctors. This book arose out of the discussion and presentations made on the day and the transcripts of the conference provided some of the material the authors needed. In particular the parents who contributed have been quoted extensively, and we are immensely grateful to them for sharing their own experiences so openly.

It may seem curious to some readers that an Academic Department of Psychiatry should have hosted a meeting for parents, clergy and doctors to share ideas in what is sometimes called the softer end of medical practice. Some colleagues in psychiatry and psychology came to the day only out of a sense of loyalty to the organisers. More than one said, 'This is not my kind of event,' but later admitted they would not have missed the day for anything!

This book endeavours to share with a wider audience some

of the insights gained from the St George's Conference. Lack of hard scientific evidence for the human needs described in these pages has not deterred the authors from exploring these softer issues even further. Those who already offer pastoral care to people with mental handicaps have perforce acquired an expertise which commands respect and deserves a wider hearing.

ONE

What's Wrong?

'How did you first discover that there was something wrong?' Many sorts of individuals can find themselves offering pastoral care to people with severe learning difficulties or to their families. Some work within church structures and are such people as clergy, parishioners or members of religious communities; others are health personnel like doctors, nurses, ancillary workers or health visitors; yet others belong to the different caring professions and are such people as social workers, counsellors, teachers, personnel officers or community workers. All of these individual carers have their own expertise; for the sake of brevity they are often collectively referred to in this book as pastoral workers. Again and again pastoral workers remark that it is impossible to have anything but a very superficial relationship with families of people with severe learning difficulties without mention being made of the way parents first became aware of their child's handicap.

Hearing the news

Often the topic is brought up spontaneously by parents, as an important part of explaining themselves and their attitude to their son or daughter. In other cases the person offering pastoral care asks how the news was broken and so indicates willingness to listen and understand this significant piece of family history. Either way the relationship between parent and pastoral worker often seems to take on greater depth once this story has been shared.

Some parents realize at once that something is amiss: 'The great moment of birth came and there was silence . . . I asked why my baby was not crying, not in my arms.'

To some the realization comes gradually:

Although in retrospect I could see that Louise did not move, smile or seem to recognize anything, I refused to see that there was anything wrong and concentrated on feeding her. Towards the end of the summer some people hinted things but I wouldn't listen. She couldn't hold her head up even but I just couldn't see anything wrong . . .

Gradually, however, we did realize that there was something terribly wrong and, as Louise was so unwell, coughing constantly, we went to see her consultant. This was in December when Louise was nine months old. We were told that Louise had had a haemorrhage as a result of her birth and that it was so severe that we should not really expect her to do anything. We were shattered, stunned, angry, and I felt foolish in that I had not seemed to notice anything wrong.

Some families find their normal child struck by sudden illness or accident, and acquired brain damage renders the normal child abnormal:

We went into intensive care. He looked so tiny, wired up to all those complicated machines. The nurses were busy doing things we didn't understand. We felt large and in the way. It was hard to believe he was the same boy that was running about full of life just a few hours before. Even before the doctor told us, somehow we knew that the old Donald had gone for ever.

Breaking the news

There is remarkable agreement among parents that they should be told the truth as soon as a diagnosis of disability or impairment is made. Ideally parents will be together. They will be in a private place, and be treated with sympathy and without hurry. They need to feel free to ask questions. Their sense of numbness, shock and inner turmoil may prevent them from hearing or understanding much of what is said, so medical staff will be prepared to repeat it as often as necessary. It has been helpful for a trusted person like a priest, hospital chaplain, social worker or friend to be with parents when they are told the diagnosis so as to help them later to recall what was said.

Certainly they will need friends, relatives and pastoral workers to be with them in the next days, weeks and months, and to listen as they struggle to make sense of what has happened. If these ideal conditions have not been met, pastoral workers will need to absorb some of the resulting anger and bitterness as well as helping parents through their mourning and grief towards acceptance.

What went wrong?

What has happened? Could it have been prevented or spotted sooner? Parents-to-be expect a normal baby to be born, and medical science is widely, although wrongly, believed to have perfected this certainty. There have been some spectacular results from putting scientific discoveries into practice. For example, in Switzerland fifty years ago the introduction of iodine to table salt reduced the incidence of mental handicap by 20 per cent by preventing hypothyroidism (cretinism). In 1953 a dietary treatment for an inherited disease called phenylketonuria was discovered which prevented the development of mental handicap. It was not until 1961 that an effective blood test was developed by Guthrie to screen all new-born babies for phenylketonuria, so that dietary treatment could be started before too much brain damage had been caused. This test is routinely done in post-natal wards around the world.

Other important advances in prevention include improved pre-natal care, better infant nutrition, the protection of infants and children by special restraints in motor vehicles and the reduction in the use of lead paint in domestic buildings. Pre-conceptual and pre-natal advice and information discourages the use of cigarettes and alcohol. If such health education becomes truly effective in the future we can expect to reduce the birth of children of low weight to mothers who smoke, and of children with foetal alcohol syndrome to those who drink.

Screening

The offer of pre-natal diagnosis is not a guarantee that all developmental disorders and genetic abnormalities will be identified. Despite an increase in the number of foetuses aborted for conditions such as Down's syndrome or neural tube defect (spina bifida), the number of children growing up with severe learning difficulties has not been greatly reduced. In part this is due to the energetic and successful resuscitation of many premature babies in neo-natal units with an associated increase in the number of children with cerebral palsy.

Present screening methods can detect only a few congenital or genetic diseases. For example, amniocentesis is a procedure routinely offered to older expectant mothers. A sample of the amniotic fluid which surrounds the foetus in the womb is removed for testing at about sixteen weeks into the pregnancy.

With this technique the timing of pre-natal diagnosis is relatively late, and if termination of the pregnancy is accepted by the parents it has to be done as soon as possible both to comply with the law, and to reduce pain and distress for the mother. With the newer diagnostic technique of chorionic villus sampling, it is possible to identify some disabling conditions as early as eight weeks.

Tissue which has the same genetic make up as the baby's — the chorionic villus that surrounds the foetus — is removed from the womb. Then this is examined in the laboratory for faulty genes. It is expected that serious genetic disorders such as thalassaemia, cystic fibrosis (the commonest genetic disease in Britain), Huntingdon's chorea and haemophilia as well as Down's syndrome and Fragile X syndrome will eventually be pinpointed by this technique. Used in conjunction with a blood test which detects a wide range of genetic diseases, a broad screening can be completed in less than an hour.

Pre-natal diagnosis is usually linked to termination of pregnancy. If the mother says she will not consider termination, perhaps for religious reasons, then pre-natal diagnosis is not offered either. When a serious abnormality is diagnosed by pre-natal screening, many parents complain that they are given inadequate information and counselling, and feel rushed into a decision which may be the most important decision of their lives. When they are given enough time to explore their feelings, to seek answers to all their questions and to weigh up the pros and cons for themselves, some parents decide to continue with the pregnancy.

When George and Jane were told that the child they were carrying had Down's syndrome, they sought extra information about the condition from the Down's Children's Association. After considering their child's future carefully they decided against a termination. Another parent was introduced to them and offered them support and comfort during the remainder of the pregnancy. Sadly their baby had congenital heart defects and was still-born.

Is information enough?

Older parents who already know about their increased risk of having a child with Down's syndrome may seek detailed information themselves before conception or before consenting to pre-natal diagnosis. We would like to see both parents offered counselling at the time pre-natal diagnosis is offered, and again when a positive diagnosis of a disabling condition has been made. Such counselling should include accurate information including access to written information about parent organizations such as the Royal Society for Mentally Handicapped Children and Adults or the Down's Children's Association, or other relevant organization. Information is not enough however, as the emotional reaction to the news will mirror the reaction when the news of handicap is broken after the child is born.

The same guidelines apply. The news should be broken to both parents together. Expression of emotional distress should be encouraged and feelings of denial, anger and rejection understood. A second interview should be offered within a day or two, and parents given another opportunity to ask questions, and to talk through their feelings. The counsellor should support the parents while they make their own decision and not impose his or her own opinion, nor encourage undue haste in the decision-making process. This is a major decision — perhaps the most important one a couple will have to make together.

With more accurate knowledge about the condition concerned and the help which would be available, parents should feel more in control and better able to cope with whichever decision they finally make. Pastoral workers who generously give time to be with parents as they struggle with such a decision can help them give voice to what they have been told and so help them rehearse the pros and cons such a decision involves. Whatever the outcome, their emotional response to losing their child, or coming to terms with a child who is different from the one they had hoped for, may require ongoing support or counselling.

This is not to deny that the birth of a child with special needs is sad news. Pre-natal diagnosis could be used more creatively to help and counsel parents, preparing them for the birth of a child who is expected to be different in one way or another.

Unfortunately, eliminating individuals who are disabled at this early stage of life devalues the status of those who remain. It does nothing to enhance our acceptance and welcome of people with mental handicap in our midst. It gives to their parents an extra burden of guilt, because 'children like that don't have to be born nowadays'.

One group of medical students at St George's Hospital Medical School joined the mental handicap course immediately after studying obstetrics. The first afternoon of the course is a light-hearted drama workshop introduced by the Strathcona Theatre Company whose members all have learning difficulties. In the discussion at the end the students questioned with amazement if these people (who mostly had Down's syndrome) were the same as the Down's syndrome foetuses they had been taught to abort.

Mourning what is lost

After parents realize that their child is handicapped their first task is to mourn the perfect child that never was or is no longer, all the hopes and aspirations that will never be realized, all the attributes taken for granted and now cruelly stripped away.

My next thoughts were for my husband, Chris. He had been told that he had a son, before the kindly nurse had realized that there was anything wrong. I knew in his mind's eye he would have already bought him rugby boots and a train set. He had to be told.

We were both unprepared for Louise. Our expectation was for normal healthy children. We had no experience of handicap. In my nursing and midwifery training I too had been geared for success.

This work of grieving for the perfect child that does not exist is not finally completed around the time of diagnosis. Every milestone can trigger off a regret for what might have been. Louise's father describes her fifth birthday:

It was actually a day we had been dreading. If Louise had been normal she would have walked to the village school with Theo and come back with her own friends and riotously torn the house apart during the party.

Learning about mental handicap

Most parents have very little knowledge of the conditions which cause severe learning difficulties. Many regard these, like traffic accidents, as liable to happen to others but not to them, while some parents can remember an individual with mental handicaps from their past and assume that their newly diagnosed child must have the same attributes.

I thought of a Mongol girl who used to hang around our village. She was always dressed in ill-fitting clothes. The thought of this girl began to haunt me when I knew that Jennifer was a Down's baby. It took me months to realize that at least there was no reason why I couldn't buy Jennifer clothes that fit her perfectly.

Parents need to find out reliable facts about their child's condition. What is mental handicap? This depends upon who is defining it.

Medical definition

The most recent and most widely used definitions of mental handicap were written by the American Psychiatric Association:[1]

A Significantly sub-average intellectual functioning: an IQ of 70 or below on an individually administered IQ test (for infants, a clinical judgement of significant sub-average intellectual functioning).

B Concurrent deficits or impairments in adaptive behaviour taking the person's age into consideration.

C Onset of the intellectual impairment before the age of eighteen years.

This definition allows for four categories of mental handicap reflecting different degrees of intellectual impairment:

Category of mental handicap	Intellectual impairment as IQ	Approximate prevalence in the population
Mild	50 — 70	30 / 1000
Moderate	35 — 49 ⎫	
Severe	20 — 34 ⎭	3.0 / 1000
Profound	below 20	0.5 / 1000

Educational definition

The Education Act 1981[2] abandoned the definition of handicap in favour of a requirement to state if a child has special educational needs. The continuum of special educational need embraces children with significant learning difficulties and emotional or behavioural disorders as well as those with disabilities of mind or body. In practice teachers had found that the causes of children's difficulties were rather complex, and that it was not possible to classify children within a single handicap category. The needs-based approach brings together a multifaceted assessment of an individual with social, educational, psychological and medical reports. The 'statement' of the child's special educational need arises from this assessment and indicates what special provision is required and why.

Legal definition

The Mental Health Act 1983[3] removed from psychiatrists the power to admit someone to hospital compulsorily simply because of his or her mental handicap (defined in the Mental Health Act 1959 as arrested or incomplete development of mind). Instead it introduced two new categories, one of which must be satisfied before compulsory hospital admission can be pursued.

Severe mental impairment means a state of arrested or incomplete development of mind which includes severe impairment of intelligence and social functioning and is associated with abnormally aggressive or seriously irresponsible conduct on the part of the person concerned.

Mental impairment means a state of arrested or incomplete development of mind (not amounting to severe mental impairment) which includes significant impairment of intelligence and social functioning and is associated with abnormally aggressive or seriously irresponsible conduct on the part of the person concerned.

Thus within the legal framework no reference is made to an individual's intellectual or educational attainments. Psychiatrists are asked to define more clearly the presence of a mental illness or behavioural problem in a person with mental handicap, and to assess the risk of any abnormally aggressive or seriously irresponsible conduct.

The intellectual impairment referred to in these definitions is permanent for any individual. Part of the pain for parents who have just heard that their child is mentally handicapped is coming to terms with the fact that this is not an illness and that he or she will never 'get better'. Yet these definitions tell us very little about what individual people can actually do or what their personality will be. It is important to remember that, whatever the degree of handicap, learning is still possible.

How common is mental illness?

There have been a number of attempts to quantify the occurrence of mental illness and behaviour disorder in people defined as mentally handicapped. The results vary widely but seem to point to the likelihood of between one and two in every five adults having a psychiatric or behavioural disturbance. If such emotional disturbance is difficult to define and quantify, it is also difficult to describe. Research is continuing to try to understand the causes of mental illness and problem behaviour and to improve our ability to recognize the signs that something is wrong and to define what is wrong. Just as a person of normal intelligence may become anxious or irritable from time to time, so may people with mental handicap. The boundary between what is normal behaviour and what is seen as abnormal will vary from one setting to another.

If a person with mental handicap also suffers from mental illness, it is clear that this may indeed get better with adequate diagnosis and treatment. Our experience is that much bizarre or antisocial behaviour among people with mental handicap can be avoided when their need for a truly personal approach to their care is understood.

Parents will want to know about their individual child's condition, its cause, its extent, its management, its prognosis. Some parents set about discovering this information with a great deal of energy, others need to be encouraged to understand and talk over the facts. For many the search for knowledge is very frustrating, abounding in false trails, false hopes and dead ends. Helpful pastors are those who say such things as:

'I don't know. Let's think where we could find out.'

'What did the specialist say? Why don't you ask again?'

'Have you talked to Zelda? She's met this situation at first hand. I'll introduce you if you like.'

'There's a self-help organization of parents like yourselves. Here's their telephone number.'

The questions parents ask may or may not have factual answers. Some information may be difficult to find because of the rarity of the disabling condition. Ann Worthington started *In Touch* some years ago for this reason. 'Contact A Family' have just launched Contact Line—a telephone information service to put callers in touch with information, support and other help.

Parents' need for information is not satisfied by answers to initial questions at the time of diagnosis. For example, when

Louise was one year old her parents were beginning to realize the full extent of her handicap. They felt very alone. On being asked if they knew what the local school was like, her father replied: 'You don't seem to understand, Louise will never go to school, never sit up, or feed herself. We will be her carers all day, every day, for the rest of her life.' No one had thought to tell them that there would be some special help.

This need for a continuous source of information persists into adult life. For example, brothers and sisters will have questions which they may want to ask about the cause of the disability. Is it hereditary? Are their children at risk of suffering the same condition? This information will have to be updated to take into account each child's changing ability to understand.

Jane's brother Andrew has the Fragile X syndrome. One effect of this inherited condition has been a severe delay in the development of his communication skills. Andrew is frustrated by his inability to think and communicate and is a difficult and unpredictable person to live with. Jane's mother sought genetic counselling for herself, her sisters and Jane to know which of them were carriers of the affected chromosome. Jane had the blood test when she was six years old and her mother tried to explain what the test meant. Her mother was carrying the affected chromosome and had transmitted it to Andrew, but Jane was not a carrier. This disorder does not have a handicapping effect on girls and women — only on boys and men. When Jane was eight she explained her understanding of the blood test and its result: 'Andrew was born before me and he has these difficulties. The blood test was to see if I was the same.' She was asked, 'Do you mean you could become like Andrew and have the same difficulties?' Jane replied that she could. She did not remember if the test was positive or negative, and she had not understood that the condition could not affect her personally.

Acknowledging the new person

Once the diagnosis is made the person receives a label which may stick for a lifetime. Right from this moment pastoral workers can help to ensure that the person is more important than the label. Use their name when referring to them: 'Simon Jones' seems more of a person than 'that handicapped Jones boy'. Interact directly with the person; hold a baby's hand and talk to him even if you get no reaction, comment on his clothes and his surroundings. Do the same to an older child with suddenly acquired brain damage. Homely, personal words and gestures show those around that this is indeed an individual.

A kind of bereavement

Most pastoral workers are familiar with the concept of bereavement stages, which are described in the classic work by Colin Murray Parkes.[4] These are not clearly distinct and to a certain extent they overlap, but the stages come in a predictable sequence and at any one time feelings from one particular stage are uppermost. Some stages may be more prolonged for certain individuals than for others. Later, at times of stress or in response to memories, the whole bereavement cycle may be triggered off again.

Pastoral workers will recognize the need to 'stay with' a bereaved person to help them work through the particular stage they have reached. Avoiding this work can cause a bereaved person to take unresolved feelings into the future, where they can distort the person's attitudes and behaviour and sap their energy. This work well done enables a bereaved person to progress towards acceptance of the loss and a resumption of ordinary living.

Bereavement work with parents whose child has mental handicaps differs from Parkes's classical work in response to loss because the child is continually present, a reminder of what might have been and a cause of extra work and worry. Such parents have a twofold task: to let go their hoped-for child and to accept another who may seem much less lovable.

If pastoral workers can identify the stages towards this acceptance they can more readily 'stay with' parents who have newly learned that their child will have severe learning difficulties. Pastoral workers are less inclined to jolly parents along or to intervene inappropriately if they listen to the things such parents typically say at nine successive stages:[5]

1. *I can't take it in.* What's happening? What are you telling me? I'm dumbfounded, lost, at sea . . .

2. *I can't cope.* I couldn't possibly take on a handicapped child. I never was any good with people like that. Help me, help me. Oh God!

3. *It's not true.* We've always been so healthy in our family. The doctor doesn't know what she's talking about. She can't be my baby, they've made a mistake. God wouldn't let it happen.

4. *It is true and I'm heartbroken.* I can't sleep. I sob so much my ribs ache and I sit rocking to and fro. To think this has happened to us. To think that God allows such things.

5. *I blame others.* It's the doctor's fault, the nurses' fault, the hospital's fault. It's all because of my husband's uncle, my wife's grandmother. I hate God for letting such things happen. I can't believe in God any more.

6. *I blame myself.* I should have known my family was tainted. I should never have decided to start this baby. I should have had a scan. I shouldn't have taken that medicine. I deserve this. God is punishing me.

7. *There's no point.* It's all hopeless. Nobody understands. The future's just a blank. How can there be a God? God can't help me.

8. *Perhaps* . . . Maybe we can cope if only he can walk and talk. Just so long as she's clean and dry. Please, God . . .

9. *Let's get on.* Let's find out what help we can get. I wonder if services exist in our area. Let's talk to other parents. Let's go to the self-help group. Let's do God's will day by day.

The bereavement process and the pastoral worker

Pastoral workers can be alert for family members to work through these stages at different rates.[6] Often a mother spends all day with her child and can negotiate these stages before her husband, who has to earn a living and keep the rest of the household going. Parents may be so absorbed in their own emotions that they forget to explain to their other children what has happened. Why is Mum so upset? What's different about our baby? Why does our baby stay in hospital, or keep going back? Have I done anything to make all this happen? Why is it all different from the way Mum said it would be? Preoccupied parents may not think of the need of their other children to deal with such questions, and may find their behaviour and emotions disturbed just when the family needs them to be 'good'. Grandparents may take much longer to come to terms with a grandchild with severe learning difficulties, and this may cause a rift between them and the child's parents. Pastoral workers who understand the bereavement process find it easier to recognize where people are and to stay with them there.

Some people show feelings more than others. Men typically find it harder to express their feelings, and may displace them on to their work or withdraw from the whole domestic situation. A sensitive pastoral worker can help a man to recognize and own some of these feelings, so that the grieving process may eventually be successfully worked through.

People go back and forth in the bereavement process, and a person who on a good day may have reached the stage of thinking they can cope, may easily slip back into going over and over whether it was their own fault or someone else's. Gradually, however, it is possible for a pastoral worker to get them to reflect that their feelings have indeed changed, that progress has been made, that they have started to 'come through'.

Sometimes pastoral workers can mobilize others to approach a grieving family and can show them what attitude is currently helpful. Often a pastoral worker can listen to parents smarting from the reactions of others. This was one mother's experience:

Chris and I were both surprised at how important other people's responses were to us. We would remember them and share them with each other. There was the dismissive, 'Oh, he won't live long then', or, 'It's for the best, isn't it dear?' These comments rated almost as low as those who immediately changed the subject. Unfortunately, people do not realize that it doesn't matter how gauche or clumsy they are in their response, so long as it is warm and sincere.

A hospital chaplain agrees:

> The bits of the New Testament I most value in a way are those when the disciples are exploring with Jesus, 'What are we going to say when hauled in front of the magistrate?' Jesus will never give too much of a rehearsed speech. He will say, 'You will know what you have to say' . . . Very often the feeling gets across rather than the words.

This chaplain went on to tell a story against himself. A little boy was having fluid drained from his brain by a shunt and this became blocked after a fall. His mother was overwhelmed by her family piling false reassurance upon her. The chaplain took her aside and said, 'Oh dear, you needed that reassurance like a hole in the head.' Then he realized what he had said. How inept, how clumsy! How could he have been so insensitive? The mother looked at him. 'Yes, you could say that, couldn't you?' she said. The chaplain concludes: 'It is very important to remember that the way in which things are said is very much more important than the words.'

One mother emphasized how greatly she and her husband needed reassurance:

> I then remember asking what I had done wrong. It must be my fault, something I had done, eaten, some drug. I was reassured then and again and again during the next week that this was not so, and for this I was immensely grateful . . . I was desperate to be told again and again, what I first learned at my parents' knee, that God loved me and God would help me. I knew these basic facts so well but I needed to be told them again, and above all by religious people.

Why do such things happen?

A child with severe learning difficulties inevitably prompts

anew the question 'Why?' H. S. Kushner grapples with this
question in *When Bad Things Happen to Good People.*[7]

A paediatrician meets it this way:

> When parents ask me why has this terrible thing happened
> to them I always shrug my shoulders and say, 'Well, I don't
> know.' That is honestly how I feel. I have no idea why these
> things happen. I usually say it is like an accident that has
> happened, there is no one at fault and this sort of thing
> always happens to someone else, never to you. Usually
> parents say that is exactly how they feel. That is probably
> how all of us feel, these kind of things never happen to us,
> they always happen to other people.

The hospital chaplain sees the question as an opportunity
to dispel mistaken and enslaving notions:

> One of my jobs as chaplain is, funnily enough, to knock
> heresy on the head. All the heresies that were around in the
> early Church are alive and well around hospitals. 'Suffering
> is good for you'—that is not Christian at all; it is nonsense.
> Parents ask, 'Am I being punished?' This always puts me
> as priest or chaplain on the line, because to believe that
> would presuppose the existence of some dreadful Fascist
> Father-God. Equally one has to take the feeling seriously.
> For what it is worth, I tend to say, 'No, I don't for one
> moment think you are being punished but it surely feels
> like it, doesn't it?'
>   One mother felt that God was punishing her. I think we
> are actually in the business of helping people to think
> religiously and we—all of us—have those magical
> connections, imagining it is because of something we have
> done. It is very, very human. I think the task of religion is
> actually to be able to tell the story so that one can unmake
> the connections. I think the greatest ministry of Jesus in the
> New Testament is the ministry of healing, in that he is the
> great disconnecter. When people say, 'This man is blind
> because he or his parents sinned,' Jesus says, 'Forget it.' He
> disconnects it. I think the disconnecting of things in the
> past with things in the present, and being able to do it
> properly, is the difference between what I think the religious
> search is all about and what I happen to think magic is all
> about.

Summary

Pastoral care for those with severe learning difficulties and their families can be offered by many sorts of people, from many different backgrounds, experiences and disciplines, each with a different contribution to make. Both at the time of diagnosis and subsequently all can play their part in helping parents to mourn their hoped-for child and to accept their child with mental handicaps. Professor Joan Bicknell gives this definition of acceptance: 'Acceptance is the death of an imaginary ideal child, and the redirection of parental love to the newly perceived child as he is in reality.' It is to this reality that we turn in the next chapter.

Notes

1. *Diagnostic and Statistical Manual*, DSM 111. American Psychiatric Association 1980.
2. Education Act 1981. HMSO.
3. Mental Health Act 1983. HMSO.
4. C. Murray Parkes, *Bereavement — Studies of Grief in Adult Life.* Penguin 1986.
5. D. J. Bicknell, 'The Psychopathology of Handicap', Inaugural Lecture, 19 November 1980 (*British Journal of Medical Psychology*, 56, 1983), pp. 167—78.
6. S. Hollins, 'Families and Handicap', in Craft, Bicknell and Hollins (ed.), *Mental Handicap.* Bailliere Tyndall 1985.
7. H. S. Kushner, *When Bad Things Happen to Good People.* Pan Books 1982.

TWO

Going Nowhere?

'When Matthew's 18 he's going to university,' proclaimed the Mencap poster, 'When Kevin's 18 he's going nowhere.' They were photographed side by side. Matthew was a bright-eyed eight-year-old, kneeling upright, arm round Kevin's shoulders. Kevin, the same age, sat cross-legged beside him. Kevin obviously had a mental handicap. The poster was produced in black and white, as if to underline the tragedy of the contrast.

Doubtless many public hearts were wrung and generous hands dipped deep into pockets. Doubtless several people stayed to read the final slogan, which was: 'More education will give Kevin more of a future.' Certainly the poster makers and sponsors intended to fund better educational chances for people with mental handicaps, and especially for the young adults. Pastoral workers can only applaud their intention, for such provision is sorely needed. Yet the poster left a lasting impression that people with mental handicaps are helpless and hopeless.

'When Kevin's 18 he's going nowhere.' What can such a poster say to the mother of a handicapped child, already fearful of the future? What does it mean to a young woman with Down's syndrome who laboriously spells out its message? What encouragement can it give to a young man with mental handicaps who cannot read but asks to have the slogan read out to him as he enters the Gateway club? Is it helpful to promote such a negative message?

This book is called 'Going Somewhere', as a reminder to those with pastoral care for people with severe learning difficulties to remain positive. It is easy to cast a person with mental handicaps as a perpetual victim, always receiving care and concern, never with anything to give. It is easy to forget anyone's need for self-esteem and self-worth, but it is even easier if the person has no speech, behaves oddly and makes very few decisions. This chapter highlights some of the ways in which Kevin tends to be treated which Matthew will probably avoid. It also suggests how Kevin might feel about his situation.

Separation from parents

Bowlby's classic study, *Child Care and the Growth of Love,*[1] was a summary of a report he wrote in 1951 under the auspices of the World Health Organization. He collated expert opinion from around the world on the subject of maternal care and mental health. He reviewed the evidence for the effect on children of a lack of personal attention and showed how young children suffer when separated from their mother or mother figure. One of the important studies he reported was Robertson's series of observations of children aged between 1 and 4 years who were undergoing separation experiences in more or less depriving institutional settings. He described three phases of response to the disruption of the attachment a child has with his mother. The first is one of protest and acute distress. The second phase is one of despair and increasing hopelessness and withdrawal. Finally the last phase is one of detachment in which the child appears to 'settle down' and accepts substitute mothering. In recognizing that the attachment between mother and child needs to be sustained rather than disrupted, care is now taken for mothers to stay in hospital with their young children.

Given Bowlby's findings it may be surprising that short-term care in hospitals, units, hostels or homes is quite often recommended for children with mental handicaps. Maureen Oswin challenges this common practice. In a critical study, *They Keep Going Away,*[2] she questions whether children with handicaps are always more exhausting than other children:

> Professionals and parents are likely to promote a very negative image of children who have handicaps if they constantly emphasize the negative aspects of a handicapped child in the family and list the advantages of his going away.

But does a physically immobile handicapped child of four years old really create more problems in his family than an ordinary, demanding, active four-year-old? And does an adolescent with Down's syndrome create more worries than the normally rebellious adolescent who is studying for O-levels, agitating for a motor-bike, seeking sexual freedom, staying out late? The worries may be very different (and long-standing) with a handicapped child, but at the same time it would seem very important that the negative effects of the handicapped child on family life are kept in proportion and occasionally reviewed to see if the problems they present are grossly in excess of those presented by children who are not handicapped. When making decisions about short-term care, questions such as the following might well be asked: Would a normal two-year-old be sent away for short-term care because he was exhausting his mother by his endless repetitive questions and demands, and, if not, then why send away a handicapped two-year-old who may never speak or get into the cupboards and take out the saucepans, but who needs help with his feeding difficulties? Do adolescents who are not handicapped get sent to hostels for short-term care because they are infuriating, rebellious and a nuisance at home, and, if not, then why is it thought necessary to send away an adolescent with Down's syndrome who may, in fact, be less of a nuisance than the normal adolescent? If the burden-and-bother aspects of handicapped children are always highlighted, this may lead to decisions being taken about them which are not only unwise, but also unjust.

Pastoral workers who accept Oswin's powerful argument are less likely to fall into the trap of agreeing that children should be removed regularly from home to hospital, hostel or special unit simply because they have mental handicaps. They are more likely to admit cheerfully that all parents need a break from time to time, that this is particularly necessary at times of family stress or illness, and that it can be useful and enriching for all children to be accustomed to stay with kindly people other than the immediate family. Being away from parents is part of the growing up process and every child should be given more opportunities to do this as he or she gets older. It is particularly important to see that a child who has disabilities is not excluded from invitations to stay with such people as grandparents or friends. It is then possible to question whether hospitals, hostels and special units staffed by professionals are the best places for children with special needs to stay.

In her study of short-term residential care services for children who are mentally handicapped Oswin describes how parents and siblings can miss their child, how the child is often homesick, how information about the child's personal routine is often ignored, how the child is expected to fit into institutional routines and often lacks stimulation and kindly attention, and how the parents are often not known, nor regarded as partners. To improve the standard of short-term care Oswin sets out seventy-five guidelines of good practice, but her preference is for special short-term foster-care schemes. She describes the close co-operation between parents and foster-parents, the continuing of home routines and programmes, the personal affection between the two families. A special foster mother is quoted as saying, 'Always think of the children as being normal, as normal children with special needs and not as handicapped children,' and her foster child said, 'I have got two lovely Mums, one at home and one here.'

Foster parents need training which will give them confidence that they do know how to meet the needs of normal children and can cope with any special needs which may arise with a particular child. They also need support when parents become very dependent upon their continued help or when their affection for their foster child becomes emotionally draining. Here is a new aspect of pastoral care. Of course, it is not argued that well-supported foster parents should replace all other forms of short-term care, but they can add considerably to the range of options presently available to hard-pressed parents.

All parents are under some kind of pressure, but for some the strain is of a different order. Some whose children, in addition to their mental handicaps, are hyperactive or have severely disturbed behaviour, or who are immobile or multiply handicapped, are among those parents who scarcely get a night's sleep. Such parents need many types of help, both within the home and outside of it, if it is to remain at all feasible for them to continue to care for their child within the community and for the child to experience the stability that this can bring. Yet these are the very children whose booked respite care is sometimes cancelled at short notice when staff sicknesses in the hostel or children's home means the staff cannot cope with the additional challenge they present, nor are these the first children to be offered shared care in another family.

> Raymond drives us to distraction. We have to put everything away. He climbs all over the furniture and uses the sofa as a trampoline. All his toys are broken. It's not fair on the other children. They can't invite friends home or keep anything precious. He loves playing with water and keeps turning the tap on. Last week our stair carpet was ruined when he left the tap running all day with the plug in. He hasn't had short-term care at the hostel for nine months now—its supposed to be one week every six. He's getting so big now (age ten) and last time he went in, he scratched a little girl badly.

This family are devoted to their son's care and very much want to be able to cope on their own. But both parents now have back trouble. They desperately need to share his care with someone.

Frequent moves

As many as 80 per cent of children with learning difficulties remain within their families, and over 50 per cent of adults remain out of long-stay care. Yet some young adults have experienced many moves, with consequent bewilderment and breaking of friendships. One man of thirty-six remembers seven such moves in his life:

> I used to live at home with my Dad. I used to get his paper for him every day from the shop. One day he said, 'You won't need to do that no more,' and I was taken to a children's home. How would you like that? I didn't do it wrong or anything. There they were quite kind to me but I left after I had fits. The next place was all right, but I

quarrelled with someone on the bus so I had to go. Then there was a hospital—I didn't like it there, the staff called me a mental defective. Well, how would you like it? Another patient said, 'Let's throw water over that fellow while he's lying in his bed,' and we did. So I had to move. The next place was all right but there was nothing much to do there. I had a friend, Pete, but I lost him when he went home again. I used to go with Phil after that but the staff said we were too much trouble and I moved again. That place was better, it was a smaller hostel and we had rooms with only two people in them. I spent most of the evenings watching telly, nothing much happened. Then my social worker said they were opening up this new home and I could ask to go there. So I did. It's the best place I've been in so far. More interesting. But I'd rather have a place of my own.

This man tends to blame himself for all the earlier moves from one placement to the next. Yet now he shows himself capable of choice and of assessing his situation. His experience exemplifies the need for pastoral workers to spend time helping people with learning difficulties to understand the reasons for such moves and to mourn the inevitable losses as well as embracing the gains. Health and local authorities are now setting up small units to prepare people living in long-stay hospitals to return to the community from which they originated. In the process lifelong friends may be parted. If such partings are inevitable, and they may not be, ways must be found to understand and express the grief felt. Here perhaps is a role for hospital chaplains and for others with pastoral care.

The effect of labelling and testing

Margaret Flynn and Christina Knussen[3] have recorded a conversation with a middle-aged woman which shows the effect upon her self-esteem of testing and labelling:

I'm a mencap. Is that the same as being mentally ill? Because when I was seventeen my mother was told I had a mental age of nine. I was with her. I'll always think like a child even though I'm forty-four . . . And the psychologist, not long ago, said about my IQ [drawing a bell shape in the air] normal people are just here, but you're below it, here.

Flynn and Knussen point out that it is more appropriate to discuss performance on a test in terms of particular strengths and weaknesses. Pastoral workers can attempt to obtain such information from testers rather than accepting uninformative total scores, and discussion about and with people with mental handicaps can proceed on the basis of their strengths. This woman also went to an Adult Training Centre where staff audibly distinguished between their 'high-grade' and 'low-grade' clients. Such labels are bound to affect both her own self-image and her attitudes to her peers, and pastoral workers need not acquiesce in their use. Flynn and Knussen refer to her throughout as 'Miss Williams': this may seem unnecessarily formal until one realizes that some people with mental handicaps are so rarely accorded the dignity of being addressed in this way that they have not learned to recognize themselves under this form of address; 'Mr Jones — that's not me, that's my father,' said one 35-year-old man with learning difficulties. If pastoral workers sometimes choose the formal form of address it can give people with mental handicaps dignity in their own eyes and in those of others.

Working through grief

One new community home faced up to the feeling of grief, loss and disparagement which seemed just below the surface for so many of the eight residents:[4]

Staff and residents met together as part of a seven-week homelife course on sexuality and relationships within the home. This particular evening they looked together at powerful black and white drawings sometimes used in bereavement counselling. The picture of a lonely young man looking on as a loving couple walk hand in hand triggered disclosures of grief and loss from staff and residents: sorrow at the death of relatives or pets; grief at leaving home or the land of one's birth; pain at apparent rejections by friends or family.

Then the staff divided up with one, two or three residents

and discussed more pictures: a boy excluded from a game of football, a dead budgie being removed from its cage, and a figure kneeling by a graveside.

We sat together for some minutes, united in shared grief. Then, since this is a Christian home, it seemed natural for one of the leaders to embrace each resident and staff-member in turn saying to each one, 'Jesus says to you today: I am with you always.' This seemed to bring relief and comfort without denying the sorrow. We had not realized that one of the leaders had inadvertently omitted to disclose a loss of her own. A resident came up to her afterwards saying, 'Haven't you got any sad things, then?'

Later staff reported greater rapport with and between the residents and with each other. When soon afterwards the mother of one of the residents died, everyone appreciated the new, mutual understanding of grief and loss.

Jean Vanier,[5] founder of the l'Arche communities, joins an intimate knowledge of the daily behaviour of people with severe mental handicaps to a unique philosophical insight. He has pondered this inner grief which he calls 'the wounded heart'. He pays tribute to the devotion and pain of parents, but continues:

It is a terrible thing for a child to feel it has let its parents down and is the cause of their pain and their tears. The wounded hearts of parents wound the heart of the child . . . Sometimes I am asked: 'Is a child or an adult who has a severe mental handicap aware of his or her condition? Do they suffer from this?' For the most part, I don't know. But this I do know: the tiniest infant senses if it is loved and wanted, or not. Similarly, people with a mental handicap, even a severe one, sense immediately whether they are loved and valued by the way they are looked at, spoken to and welcomed . . . If the little one does not sense its mother's love — which not only rejoices in her baby's beauty and uniqueness, but also in its potential for growth, for autonomy and eventual separation from her — then the baby feels lost and enters into anguish. It experiences an inner emptiness or an inner suffocation.

Vanier goes on to speak of a child

> cutting itself off from the deep feelings of the heart and
> hiding in the world of dreams. When the heart of a person
> is solidly barricaded in this way, there is psychosis. If the
> barriers are less solid, there is instability, sometimes deep
> depression, agitation, apathy or agression . . .
> When I see Evelyn banging her head against the floor . . .
> when I see Luke aimlessly running round and round . . .
> when I see the closed, tense face of George, I know in each
> there is a profound agony and an unbearable interior
> restlessness.

All human beings erect barricades, and a wounded heart is
not produced in a child only by the attitudes of parents.
There is a void within all people which can be filled by God
alone:

> The Christian doctrine on the wounded heart, or original
> sin, appears to me the one reality that is easily verified . . .
> in the heart of each of us there is division, there is fear,
> there is fragility; there is a defence system which protects
> our vulnerability, there is flight from pain, there is evil and
> there is darkness.

The wounded heart is healed through relationships of trust
with significant others, and through learning to trust God as
Jesus did:

> When a child discovers through a Christian community
> that it is possible to have a personal relationship with God,
> everything changes. It is no longer necessary to live the
> relationship with one's parents in ambivalence, expecting
> too much from them and blaming them when those
> expectations are disappointed. Even if one is sometimes
> disappointed, it is still possible to love them.

All people need trusting relationships, and with them loss
can be faced and mourned and become a source of strength:

> The particular drama of those who have a mental or
> physical handicap is that these losses come too early in life,
> before they have acquired the inner strength that would
> enable them to face loss. Sometimes loss comes at birth, or
> even during the pregnancy, when the baby is deprived of

the love and esteem of its parents, affecting physical and psychic development. These losses and the grief which follows invade the life of the child prematurely, when it has neither the strength nor the human means to cope. Moreover, sometimes the child has to face a distress so profound that it can be overcome only if there is a deep inward experience of the love of God. In that love which burns, illuminates and enlivens the heart, one discovers that one is precious to God just as one is, in one's very being. That love gives meaning to life, it gives strength to continue living; it enables the person to break out of the cycle of sorrow and anger; it stops the flight into illusion.

Summary

Kevin, and all children with learning difficulties, have potential and are 'going somewhere'. Some of their handicaps are not intrinsic but may be aggravated by short-term placements, by frequent moves and broken friendships, and by insensitive testing, classifying and labelling. Bereavement therapy can assuage these wounds, which add to the original wound sustained when children sense that they are the cause of their parents' grief. The wounded heart can only be healed by consistent relationships of trust with other people and with God.

Within Christian and other religious traditions this trusting relationship with God is important. However the issues discussed in this chapter are not met exclusively in church circles but will be relevant in all caring environments.

Notes

1. John Bowlby, *Child Care and the Growth of Love.* Penguin 1953.
2. Maureen Oswin, *They Keep Going Away.* King's Fund Publishing Office (14 Palace Court, London W2 4NT) 1984.
3. Margaret Flynn and Christina Knussen, 'What It Means to be Labelled "Mentally handicapped" ' (*Social Work Today,* 16 June 1986).
4. Rosemary McCloskey and Margaret Grimer, 'Friends and Strangers' (*Disability Now,* July 1986).
5. Jean Vanier, *Man and Woman He Made Them.* Darton, Longman and Todd 1985.

THREE

How Normal Is Normal?

Pastoral workers who start to care for people with learning difficulties soon come to realize that there are two powerful movements afoot. One is the closure of long-stay hospitals and the transfer of people with mental handicaps back into the local community. The second is the change in every setting to less institutional ways of working, offering people more choice and more self-determination. The principle underlying both these movements has come to be known as normalization.

What is normalization?

The main goal of normalization, according to its chief developer Wolf Wolfensburger, is 'to create or support socially valued roles for people in their society.'[1] At its heart is the avoidance of all that is second-rate and second-best, and of anything that tends to exclude an individual from the rest of that person's society. A distinction can be made between normalization of the individual and of the environment. Making detailed individual plans is important to help individuals to make progress in socially valued roles; a more normal environment requires the development of ordinary housing and improved access to everyday facilities.

Normalization training

Seminars are proliferating to introduce medical and care staff to the principles of normalization.

One useful resource is the Lifestyles training pack,[2] which looks at the way people with mental handicaps are valued as persons and as sexual beings, and pinpoints ways in which Kevin's life may differ from Matthew's.

Participants are given cards listing 80 circumstances which Matthew may enjoy while Kevin does not or which Kevin may be subjected to but Matthew escapes. Items include:

> being able to leave your things lying around;
> masturbating alone in private;
> needing to ask permission to marry when you are
>   thirty-five;
> being called a 'boy' or a 'girl' when you are grown up.

Participants decide which circumstances they value highly or else would wish to avoid for themselves. In this light they reflect on the lifestyles and opportunities commonly made available to people with a mental handicap. Finally they decide which changes they have the power and desire to bring about for people with mental handicaps in their care.

The Lifestyles training exercise can cause staff to face up for the first time to the fact that, if Kevin is deprived of rights that Matthew enjoys or is subjected to unwelcome treatment that Matthew escapes, this is rarely due directly to his handicaps. Far, far more often it is due either to the attitudes of others or to the services Kevin receives. The exercise is a powerful agent for change.

The same values are promoted in another excellent training pack produced jointly by Mencap and the Open University and entitled *Mental Handicap—Patterns for Living*.[3] This enables groups of parents, relatives, or those working with people with mental handicaps to understand and promote their rights, abilities and independence in many practical ways. It is valuable, too, for pastoral workers to use with church and voluntary groups.

Normalization can be a long process

Sometimes the idea of normalization is embraced unthinkingly. People with mental handicaps who used to be cared for in long-stay hospitals can be lost and exploited if they suddenly find themselves dumped without proper preparation in inner-city houses. Seeing such things done in the name of normalization has caused Elly Jansen, the founder of the

Richmond Fellowship, to say: 'Normalization is one of the dirtiest words in the book. A very uncaring attitude.'

If Kevin has never been allowed to choose what cereal he wants for breakfast he is unlikely to be able to choose whether or not he wants a long-term sexual relationship. Jenny Cooper makes this point in an article entitled, 'Remember They Are Not Normal': [4]

> What we must guard against is that when a mentally handicapped person reaches adulthood chronologically we do not run out of patience and start treating him like an adult. We cannot expect him to behave like an adult if intellectually he is still a child.
>
> He will develop but it will be that much slower and we must be that much more patient. If we try to rush his development we may be doing him more harm than good. He will feel insecure because we are not accepting him as he is — we want to change him before he is ready . . . We do need to take into account the emotional and intellectual ages of our clients. Allowing them to do just what they want may not necessarily be a caring attitude.

It is clear that adults with mental handicaps still need to be accepted exactly as they are and then to make graded progress towards greater freedom and autonomy. Normalization cannot mean leaving them to sink or swim. Properly understood it can remind pastoral workers of Kevin's years of experience, and of his rights and personal worth. It can prevent pastoral workers from complacent or despairing acquiescence in the status quo.

Helping parents to appreciate the principles of normalization

Parents of young adults with mental handicaps are now starting to undertake the Lifestyles training exercise. They are often amazed at the realization that their attitudes may be preventing their adult sons and daughters from being more independent. Some parental resolutions after doing the exercise were:

> to get rid of all my daughter's conventional kilts and

cardigans and to enlist the help of my other teenage daughters in helping her to choose more trendy clothes;

to fix the wardrobe door so that it opens the other way, making it easier for my daughter to select her own clothes in the morning;

to visit the local shop to explain that my son will be coming in later to buy his own Walkman, telling the shopkeeper what help will be needed, then leaving them to sort out the transaction together;

reminding my son to change for bed half an hour before the TV snooker programme, then putting on the programme as a reward for changing by himself;

making sure the sidesman at church understands that my daughter likes to be given a hymn book. It's not important that she can't read it. She enjoys holding a book like everybody else.

Jean Vanier's attitude to normalization

The first l'Arche communities were founded before the drive for normalization. It is a movement which Jean Vanier[5] welcomed:

A kind of revolution had begun, especially in the 1970s. People began to discover that those with a mental handicap had astonishing potential for growth, that many who had been stigmatized were able to work and live happily like everyone else.

Thus was born in the rich countries, especially in Scandinavia, the principle called 'normalization' for those with a mental handicap. According to these principles, those people with a handicap must live like everyone else; at any price, segregation must be avoided. Treat someone like a fool and that person becomes a fool. To fear someone is to instil in that person a fear of himself or herself and fear of others. Similarly, a person who is treated as 'normal' will become 'normal'.

I discovered this for myself, as I lived with men and women who had been locked up in asylums. The way you look at people can transform them.

Vanier goes on to look squarely at the questions normalization raises for sexual relationships between men and women with mental handicaps, and this is the subject of a later chapter.

Normalization as an ethical principle for society

The fact of mental handicap gives rise to many problems of ethics. Is it right or wrong to offer parents pre-natal diagnosis and subsequent abortion, or for parents to accept it? What are the limits of treatment and care? Is it right to give sexual education to a person with learning difficulties, or wrong not to? How far can a person with mental handicaps give informed consent to contraception or abortion? Can people with mental handicaps contract a valid marriage?

These are important ethical questions, and many of them are considered elsewhere in this book. We should like here to state our own ethical viewpoint, which is that all other ethical questions concerning people with mental handicaps are less important than this:

> *Do we wholeheartedly accept people with mental handicaps as full members of our society?*

Replying 'Yes' to such a question would imply working to enable people with mental handicaps to have ready access to:

1. The generic health services, like family doctor and dentist, audiologist, physiotherapist, accident and emergency departments.

2. The ordinary education services.

3. Ordinary religious and church services.

4. Ordinary clubs and societies.

5. Ordinary shops, places of entertainment, sports facilities and tourism.

6. Ordinary voluntary services.

Special services would be available to meet special needs, but only where the ordinary services and facilities cannot be adapted to meet them. People with mental handicaps would never be forced to do separately what they could do together with the rest of us.

To move nearer to this ideal, ordinary services can ask themselves these hard questions:

Do we ever refuse to serve people with mental handicaps?

Do people with mental handicaps use our service at present?

Do they have physical access?

Do they know about our service?

Do they know they would be welcome?

Do they feel welcome when they come?

Do we cater for their special needs?

Can we adapt to meet their special needs better?

Pastoral workers are often well placed to ask these questions of ordinary services. Raising consciousness is an important work which pastoral workers are in a good position to carry out.

Watch your language

The principle of normalization demands care in the way we speak of people with mental handicaps. Words are powerful. The way we describe someone affects the way we act towards them.

One example is the use of the expression 'Down's syndrome' which is the official name given to the medical syndrome chromosome 21 Trisomy, first described by Down in 1886. Many older people grew up hearing people with this condition referred to as 'Mongols'. A short word, it picks out facial characteristics which many people with this syndrome share with many people from Mongolia. Of course, it was inaccurate: most people with the syndrome do not come from Mongolia, they are of all nationalities. It carried overtones of the foreigner and the stranger, and even of the uncontrolled Mongol hordes who historically overran peaceful people, raping and pillaging as they went. More aware people with the syndrome realized that the word 'Mongol' tended to group them with other less able people, and then they were assumed to have all the disabilities ascribed to the group as a whole. The condition became a subject for academic study and its complexity began to be realized.

These factors combined to make many people feel that it was time to describe people with this condition differently, and a concerted effort was made to use the expression 'Down's syndrome'. Crusaders made it their mission to challenge the expression 'Mongol' whenever it was used; many meetings, conferences and discussions were sidetracked from the business in hand when participants inadvertently slipped into the old ways and crusaders would not allow them to continue without correction.

Labelling and classifying

This exemplifies some general principles about labels:

1. Changing a name does not change a fact. People will continue to have Down's syndrome whatever we choose to call it.

2. Labels need not be meant unkindly to have unkind effects. Those using the expression 'Mongol' did not mean to imply that people were alien or uncontrolled, but they could not prevent others from receiving such a message.

3. Precise terms can encourage accurate knowledge. Using the term 'Down's syndrome' can make me aware of what is known academically about the condition and can remind me that it is worthy of study.

4. The label I use can make a change in my attitude. Once I realize that people with Down's syndrome sometimes understand and resent my label I will not use it in their presence, and not using it can remind me to ask their opinion in other matters.

5. Changing the label can help to bring about attitude change in others. Discussions and challenges about terminology can lead to a re-evaluation of attitudes.

6. People receiving labels given to a group tend in the eyes of others to assume all the characteristics attributed to that group. A person may have slight learning difficulties but being constantly grouped with others with Down's syndrome may lead to their abilities being underestimated.

7. All labels attaching to a group with unwanted characteristics tend over time to attract a stigma. Even when such labels are originally acceptable they tend to become less so with time, and must be changed to avoid giving offence where none was previously taken.

8. Newer labels are often longer or clumsier than the old. 'Men and women with Down's syndrome' is far more of a mouthful than 'Mongols'. It requires more care to speak or write it. For such a complicated phrase, real conviction of its importance is needed to change long-standing habit.

9. Changing the terminology is difficult, but it is easier than changing attitudes and behaviour. Calling someone 'a woman with Down's syndrome' is of little help if my behaviour towards her remains overbearing or lacking in respect.

10. Any label may be used far too often. A person's name is usually far more relevant. This point is succinctly summed up by the following Down's Children's Association poster slogan: 'You say mongol, we say Down's syndrome, his mates call him David.'

People first

These general principles can be helpful to pastoral workers starting to work with people who have mental handicaps. Words like 'defective' and 'subnormal', kindly meant in their day and used to replace even more pejorative terms, today generally are understood to be words of rejection. A more acceptable term is 'handicap', which emphasizes simply the extra difficulties some people face. Handicaps are described as mental in contrast to physical, although the term 'intellectually handicapped', favoured in Australia, has much to recommend it. Exception is taken to expressions such as 'the handicapped' or 'the mentally handicapped', since here the person is defined by and lost in the group's disability, and it seems particularly insensitive to refer to people as though they actually are the condition they are affected by. The slogan 'PEOPLE FIRST' can act as a reminder to think of the person before the disability, and also to use such expressions as 'people with mental handicaps' or 'people with learning difficulties'. In fact, now that the term 'handicap' is so widely used, it may be starting to collect a certain generalized stigma and expressions like 'people with learning difficulties' are preferred by many.

It is also important to understand what messages are received when patronizing, sentimental or sensational words are used. Terms like 'unfortunates', 'poor souls', 'the helpless', 'the afflicted', 'pathetic victims' or 'sufferers' imply that life for people with learning difficulties is one long drudge. Expressions such as 'God's holy innocents' or 'eternal child' do nothing to give adult status to grown men and women with mental handicaps. Their parents are not helped by constant references to their courage, bravery, fortitude or tragedy, nor do they spend all their life struggling and battling. Saints and martyrs they may be, but only in an ordinary sense that applies to many good people. Their situation is not helped by referring to their son or daughter as a cross, a burden or a trial.

Pastoral workers can make a conscious choice to lessen their use of all these negative expressions and to start using more positive ones. Positive phrases stress justice (right, fair, due, entitled), normality (ordinary, daily, taken for granted, usual, mainstream, everyday), progress (step by step, bit by bit, little by little, come a long way, getting there), integration (accepted, belonging, part of, one of us) and autonomy (independent, choice, decision, making up your own mind).

Such care with terminology may be daunting to pastoral workers whose expertise is other than mental handicap but who occasionally see people with mental handicaps in the course of their work. The main message of the 'People First' campaign is not to define people by their handicap or to feel that expert knowledge is needed before interacting with them.

It would be sad if pastoral workers were to feel inhibited towards people with learning difficulties for fear of using the wrong phrase. In human relationships much is forgiven to people who are genuine. A useful tip is to leave out any reference to handicap or disability unless it is relevant. It is Mary who likes to collect postcards, not her mental handicap that predisposes her to do it. Swapping postcards with a mentally handicapped girl is subtly different from swapping postcards with Mary.

A progress checklist

Pastoral workers who wish to test whether they are doing everything feasible to ensure that a person with mental handicaps is offered as normal a life as possible can check their performance against these five normalizing 'accomplishments' listed by O'Brien:[6]

1. Ensure a person's presence in their own community.

2. Promote the person's individual interests, preference and choices.

3. Develop the person's skills for independent living.

4. Afford the person respect, and demand that others do the same.

5. Facilitate the person's participation in the local community.

Summary

Changes are needed in attitudes, in services and in vocabulary before people with mental handicaps are able to take their rightful places as full members of society. The most important ethical question posed by the fact of mental handicap is 'Have we the will to make these changes?'

Notes

1. W. Wolfensburger, *The Principle of Normalisation in Human Services.* Toronto National Institute on Mental Retardation 1973.
2. H. Brown and J. Alcoe, *Lifestyles for People with Mental Handicaps — a staff training exercise based on normalisation principles.* East Sussex Consultancy and Training Agency 1984.
3. Open University, *Mental Handicap: Patterns for Living,* study pack P555. 1986.
4. Jenny Cooper, 'Remember They Are Not Normal' (*Community Care,* 8 May 1986).
5. Jean Vanier, *Man and Woman He Made Them.* Darton, Longman and Todd 1985.
6. J. O'Brien and A. Tyne, *The Principle of Normalisation — a Foundation for Effective Services.* London Campaign for the Mentally Handicapped 1981.

FOUR

Sex Discovered

If normalization is rightly understood as a process, with appropriate education available at each successive stage, it can be a valuable principle for understanding sex and sexuality. The principle implies that the sexuality of people with learning difficulties is recognized and they are helped to understand and realize their sexual potential. It implies that their sexual rights are respected, and that they are offered education to be able to carry out the corresponding duties and to respect the rights of others. Often this is not easy.

People with mental handicaps are sexual persons

It seems obvious that, just as the rest of us are born male or female, so also are people with learning difficulties. Boys are born with a penis, and grow into men with seminal emissions and the possibility of having sexual intercourse with a woman and fathering a child: girls are born with a vagina, and grow into menstruating women with the possibility of having sexual intercourse with a man and bearing a child.

This may be self-evident, but the former attitude of regarding people with mental handicaps as eternal children has caused some people to think of them as asexual. Adolescence can cause a crisis for some parents who have accepted their handicapped child as a child but have not accepted that this child would become a sexually active man or woman. People who tolerate or are amused by childish behaviour can withdraw their sympathy when the actor is six feet tall and sexually fully developed.

Acceptance of the sexuality of people with handicaps can also be affected by the mass media. Where advertisements, TV programmes and magazines overwhelmingly show sexual relationships as happening between the young, the athletic

39

and the beautiful, what chance is there of finding it normal for a middle-aged woman with Down's syndrome to want a personal and sexual relationship with a man who has slight brain damage and partial paralysis?

Whose problem?

The sexuality of people with mental handicaps is often a problem for the onlooker rather than for handicapped persons themselves. They may in all innocence undress inappropriately, or show affection in the wrong way to the wrong person at the wrong time in the wrong place and before the wrong audience. This may disturb the handicapped person not at all. It is the onlooker whose sense of propriety is outraged.

Where sexuality is concerned, simple facts are never just facts and they are never simple. We all have feelings about sex, some of which seem quite respectable and which we would not mind owning, others which we would reveal only to a trusted confidant, others again which we hope nobody discovers and which we do not like to own even to ourselves. Inappropriate sexual behaviour on the part of an unaware person with learning difficulties can trigger off sexual feelings in ourselves, so that our reaction is coloured by our feelings. It is important for those with pastoral care for people with mental handicaps to get in touch with their own feelings about sexuality, so that they can recognize where these distort their judgement. One wise teacher of adolescents with learning difficulties goes by this maxim: 'Whenever there is agitation about the sexual activities of someone in my care my first rule is "Cool it!" And I know that this applies to myself just as much as to anybody else.'

How important is social acceptance?

Whatever the intentions of the person with learning difficulties, it is certain that they must be educated in the proprieties. The myth of the person with mental handicaps as uncontrolled sexual pervert is even older than that of the eternal child. Acceptance within ordinary society depends on people being able to behave respectably, and the normalization process will be greatly hindered if a person suffers rejection because of his or her inappropriate sexual behaviour. Yet it is sometimes forgotten that uncontrolled outbursts and shocking behaviour are well known in adolescents without mental handicaps.

People say, 'He's just going through a stage,' or, 'She's driving me mad. I'll be glad when she's learned some sense,' as teenagers slam doors, turn up the decibels, verbally attack their elders, lock themselves in their rooms, experiment sexually, choose wildly unsuitable partners and flout their parents' cherished beliefs. For most parents there are several uneasy years before a combination of insisting on minimal standards, turning a blind eye, offering and receiving forgiveness and picking up the pieces and trying again is transformed into an adult relationship where parents and child treat each other as equals and the adult son or daughter has achieved a freely chosen lifestyle different from that of the parents. When adolescents with learning difficulties throw plates, hit others, damage furniture, expose themselves in public, compulsively masturbate, fondle each other or try to have sexual intercourse behind the rubbish bins, somehow this is all ascribed to their mental handicap. It is forgotten how much perforce is forgiven to other adolescents. The fact that adolescents with a mental handicap need more help and enjoy less privacy means that parents have far less chance of ignoring their adolescent sexual experiments.

For some people who have very profound mental handicaps their sexuality seems almost irrelevant and their response is to bodily care and comfort, to gentle and affectionate tending. Their dignity can be enhanced by their setting, with pictures and decor suited to their age and sex, and by their clothes being specially chosen to reflect their maleness or their femininity but, for these few, sexual education may not be appropriate. For others it is vital if they are to progress towards normality.

How important is self-acceptance?

If traditional sex education was to give as little sexual information as possible, this applied even more to children with mental handicaps. No future sexual relationship was expected for them, so there was 'no need to put ideas into their heads'. Sexual training was likely to consist of 'Don't!' and 'Stop it!' and 'That's dirty!'. Commitment to normalization implies an end to this negative training.

Ann and Michael Craft[1] have for long championed the rights of people with mental handicap to a proper sexual education. Ann Craft[2] has summed up her philosophy like this:

> Sexual needs, feelings and drives are an inherent part of being human. They are not optional extras that we in our wisdom can choose to bestow or withhold according to whether or not someone passes an intelligence test. In reality the issue is how can we channel them into socially acceptable expression? What do people with mental handicaps need to know and what do they need to understand about themselves, their feelings and their behaviour which will offer them both protection and a means of enriching life?

The aim is for all people with mental handicaps to accept their own body, to understand its workings as far as they are able and to feel at ease and comfortable about it. This requires an early start and constant repetition in naming penis and scrotum for boys, vagina for girls. It requires parents to show the same pleasure in these parts of their young child's body as they show in fingers, toes, ears or noses. It requires that a child grows up with the sensual satisfaction of being touched, hugged and kissed.

Well before puberty girls need to know that they will have periods, and develop breasts and pubic hair. Routines for changing sanitary pads have to be thought out and practised, perhaps with the help of a set of colour photographs such as those published by the Jack Tizard School Consortium.[3]

A group of mothers was discussing the problem of preparing their daughters for menstruation in spite of their learning difficulties. They agreed that this education might take some time and so it would have to begin well before the periods started. They made a promise that, from their daughter's ninth birthday, they would start to talk about their own menstruation, showing the Jack Tizard pictures. The next stage was to show their own sanitary pads and how they put them on. Later they showed their soiled pads and how they disposed of them. Next they encouraged their daughter to wear sanitary pads herself whenever mother had a period, practising for having periods 'just like Mother'. When the daughter's period finally started it was greeted with delight: 'Now you have your own period at your own time. Well done!' One father celebrated the start of his daughter's period by giving her a bunch of flowers, another by presenting her with her first grown-up necklace.

Boys also need to start their sexual education early with the same gradual approach. Wendy McCarthy and Lydia Fegan[4] give a summary of what boys need to know:

1. 'Hair will grow under your arms and around your penis and then on your face. It will feel different from the hair on your head.'

2. 'Your penis and testicles will grow larger and from time to time your penis will get hard and stick up. Sometimes this will seem to happen for no reason at all: other times it will happen when you're thinking about sex or girls or when you read something in a magazine. It can be embarrassing but it happens to everyone. The word for this is erection. An erection is a private thing. Do not ask everyone to look at it. It will go away.'

3. 'Sometimes you will wake up in the morning and think you have wet the bed because all the sheets are wet and sticky. This means you have had what we call a wet dream. You haven't wet the bed—you have ejaculated some semen during the night. Wipe the semen off with tissue and wash yourself. Put your pyjamas and sheets out to wash or air if they're very messy.'

4. 'The semen that comes out of your penis has sperm in it which helps make a baby. It doesn't matter how much sperm comes out of your penis. Your body continues to make more all the time.'

5. 'It is OK to think about sex or to dream about it. Everyone does. Dreams, thoughts and fantasies won't hurt you or anyone else.'

6. 'Lots of boys feel the need to rub their penis or masturbate
    when they get an erection. That's fine. Everyone does it,
    but remember that it is a private thing, not something
    that we do in public.'

McCarthy and Fegan stress that parents should start these
explanations well before puberty and repeat them many times,
so that as the changes occur they can be greeted with positive
recognition. They also point to the general need for education
in self-reliance, good grooming and hygiene.

Is masturbation a problem?

Most people realize that masturbation of itself is not harmful;
it is part of a process of self-discovery and it gives the
individual a certain pleasure and relief from tension. Yet the
same people would like to direct adolescents and adults with
mental handicaps who are in their charge away from
masturbating in public, finding that it is embarrassing, it
makes their charges unacceptable to others and it prevents
their progress in normalization.

McCarthy and Fegan are clear that parents and carers
should teach positively that masturbation is only to be done
in private:

> Masturbation is not acceptable in the schoolroom or in the
> workplace. There is no point in ignoring it or pretending
> that it is not happening simply because you, as a parent or
> a teacher, don't know how to deal with it. Most
> intellectually handicapped people can be taught that
> masturbating is something done only at home in private
> and that it is not appropriate elsewhere. However, if they
> are not allowed to do it in private at home, they are likely to
> continue doing it in public.
>
> It may take a great deal of patience and perseverance on
> the part of parents to take their children, even as adults, to
> their room every time they start to masturbate. Stress that
> they are not being reprimanded for masturbating, only for
> doing it in the wrong place. If they can learn to distinguish
> between things people do in public and things people do in
> private, such as going to the toilet, bathing or dressing,
> they will learn the concept of privacy for masturbation.[4]

When parents or carers believe that masturbation is wrong even in private it is still possible for them to view the move from public to private masturbation as a desirable step, the first attempt to exercise some kind of self-control.

Jean Vanier[5] does not accept what he calls

the modern tendency to trivialize masturbation, saying, 'It is not important. It is normal, simply a question of adolescence. It will pass. Do not make a fuss about it . . .'

Adolescence is of crucial importance, because it is a time of growth to sexual maturity. That maturity is shown in a real commitment towards others, a commitment which is not just a running away from one's own suffering into the outside world but one which springs from inner peace, harmony and the search for unity and truth within.

Yet Vanier is full of understanding for the fragility and inner agitation which cause people to masturbate, and points to humankind's need for touch and tenderness and personal relationships:

. . . we must recognize that there are no fixed or precise laws. This is the reality of each human person and of his or her growth. In order to grow, each person needs to be surrounded by friends and be regarded as full of potential for growth.

With their more pragmatic approach McCarthy and Fegan come to a similar conclusion: 'If people are masturbating repeatedly, an attempt should be made to find out what is causing the anxiety. It may mean they need more touching and hugging and more expressions of love and affection.'

They remind parents and carers not to overlook the possibility of local irritation: 'If a girl masturbates compulsively, and seemingly without too much pleasure, it is worth checking whether she has a vaginal infection which is itchy and needs to be scratched or rubbed.'

McCarthy and Fegan are also quick to point out that often it is not learning disabilities which cause people to masturbate but lack of more interesting opportunities: 'Sometimes, if people are bored and lonely and have few stimuli around them, they tend to make masturbation a full-time distraction, in the same way as other people eat a lot or watch TV.' An hour at the swimming bath may not prevent masturbation but it certainly gives people something else to do with their bodies.

One resource that is often overlooked in the effort to direct people with mental handicaps away from masturbating in public is the influence of their peers. Often other residents at a home or hostel or other pupils at a school or trainees at an ATC can encourage someone to go to the bedroom or bathroom, and if their help is tactfully enlisted it can be the most effective intervention.

Preventing exploitation

Young children today are taught to value their bodies and to protect themselves against sexual harassment and exploitation. People with mental handicaps tend to attract more than their fair share of both.

'My body's my own' is a useful slogan for them also. Another useful exercise is the 'What if . . .?' game described by Michele Eliot:[6]

> Playing 'What if' games, either at home or in school, is a good way for children to learn many concepts. You can start with a variety of situations not related to assaults. For example:
>
> ADULT: What if you saw smoke coming from your neighbour's house?
>
> CHILD: I would ring the fire brigade.
>
> ADULT: How would you do that? Demonstrate for me.
>
> This would be a good way to teach a child about making 999 calls. Examples of preventative 'What if' games might be:
>
> ADULT: What if someone said he or she was a friend of Daddy's and asked you to go with him or her to a house?
>
> CHILD: I would not go and would run away if anyone got too close. I would tell a grown-up what happened.
>
> When the children are prepared for the more sensitive questions, ask:

ADULT: What if a babysitter or relative you liked asked you to play secret games, and offered to let you stay up late (or give you a present or money, etc.)?

CHILD: I would say that I am not allowed to keep secrets.

ADULT: What if the person insisted?

CHILD: I would say No and say I was going to tell. Then I would tell.

A catchphrase to go with this exercise is 'Just say NO'. Obviously any exercise which furthers self-image and esteem is also helpful in preventing exploitation, as is a proper degree of assertion.

Adults living in a small group home were taught how to discriminate between different callers at the door:[7]

We asked who came to the door of this home. Residents named people and we listed them in three categories; strangers who are asked to wait outside, callers who are invited to wait in the hall and friends who came right in.

We talked about how to distinguish strangers from callers. There are no Makaton signs so we devised our own symbols: an empty red circle and an amber one with 2 eyes. Each resident had a go at role playing answering the door, with much advice and laughter from the others. Our symbol for a friend was a green circle with 2 eyes and a smiling mouth. With the help of staff the residents named the friends who called and we discussed the routine for greeting friends, entertaining them and saying goodbye. There was lively role play and a slogan emerged: 'Goodbyes are short and sweet'.

Later it is possible to elaborate this teaching further, as in the system of concentric 'Circles of social distance' developed by Marklyn P. Champagne and Leslie Walker-Hirsch:[8]

At the centre is the 'purple self circle': it is appropriate to touch oneself anywhere one pleases, but nobody else has this right. Radiating outwards comes the 'blue circle' of family, boyfriend or girlfriend, where exchanges of hugs, kisses and cuddles are appropriate. Next comes the 'green circle' of friends, with their own appropriate but less intimate contact. Beyond that is the 'yellow handshake circle' for acquaintances, an 'orange wave circle' for children and at the outside a 'red circle' for strangers, who are not to touch or be touched.

The precise number of circles of social distance and the precise behaviours taught for each can be varied with different individuals and with different communities and cultures. What is important here is for pastoral workers to know that it is often possible over time to teach people with learning disabilities to recognize social and sexual distance and to learn the level of bodily intimacy appropriate for each encounter. This discrimination can greatly reduce the risk of sexual exploitation from strangers and of provocative or inappropriate sexual behaviour on the part of the person with learning difficulties. They can learn, for instance, that they should not stop and play with young, unknown children.

This kind of education is very important and cannot be started too early. Without it people with mental handicaps are liable to be exploited or to exploit others sexually. They may then have to be more closely supervised, and so their progress towards a normal life is in danger of being halted or reversed.

Summary

In spite of the difficulties this creates within parents and carers, people with mental handicaps are full sexual beings. They need education in proper social behaviour, in self-knowledge and awareness and to prepare them for puberty. Most can learn to accept their own bodies and to respect those of other people.

Notes

1. Ann and Michael Craft, *Sex Education and Counselling for Mentally Handicapped People.* Costello 1983.
2. Ann Craft, 'Sexuality and mental handicap' (*Physiotherapy,* April 1985).

3. *Coping with My Period.* ESNS Consortium. Jack Tizard School, Finlay Street, London SW6 6HB.
4. Wendy McCarthy and Lydia Fegan, *Sex Education and the Intellectually Handicapped: a Guide for Parents and Care Givers.* ADIS Press (404 Sydney Road, Balgowlah, NSW 2013, Australia) 1984.
5. Jean Vanier, *Man and Woman He Made Them.* Darton, Longman and Todd 1985.
6. Michele Eliot, *Preventing Child Sexual Assault.* Bedford Square Press (26 Bedford Square, London WC1B 3HU) 1985.
7. Rosemary McCloskey and Margaret Grimer, 'Friends and Strangers' (*Disability Now*, July 1986).
8. Marklyn P. Champagne and Leslie Walker-Hirsch, *Circles* (a two part sound/slide series with accompanying 5' x 5' wall graphic). James Stanfield Publishing Company, PO Box 1983—C, Santa Monica, CA 90406, USA.

FIVE

Relationships: Sexual or Personal?

Some of the most vocal advocates of rights for handicapped people are very clear that this includes the right to sexual relationships. Such relationships are sometimes recommended as a relief from sexual frustration, or as an assertion of equality. It is our belief that sexual intercourse by itself can never satisfy a person's longing for love, for belonging, for acceptance and for significance. When sexual intercourse happens as part of a loving relationship it can signify and affirm all of those things. Without a loving relationship it is more likely to lead to a feeling of disillusion and failure or of being exploited and used. For this reason we consider it irresponsible for parents and carers to encourage people with mental handicap to have a sexual relationship unless there is already a reasonable personal relationship between the partners and they are prepared to foster this and give the couple every chance to develop it.

People with mental handicaps do sometimes have sexual intercourse casually or without love just as other people do. Then it is for parents and pastors to stand by and be ready to pick up the pieces.

How important are loving relationships?

With or without sexual intercourse, relationships of love can be very important to men and women with mental handicaps, as they are to us all. To feel accepted, wanted and understood, to have a partner to share experiences with, this is precious indeed. A way of being intimate which involves hugging, kissing, holding hands and sharing is worthwhile even if a particular man and woman are not interested in having sexual intercourse.

For such a couple to be able to share a room in a hostel or

group home requires changes of attitude on the part of staff and other residents. For such a couple to set up home together successfully requires that they have enough insight to understand and respond to each other's needs and some of the skills of independent living. Both call for careful preparation.

Apart from any one particular relationship, people with mental handicaps depend like us all upon a network of friends to give them a sense of well-being and significance.

Is marriage possible?

Of the population as a whole, 95 per cent marry, but very few people with a mental handicap do so at present. Miss Williams, whose observations on being classified as mentally handicapped have been quoted previously, obviously thought marriage was not for her: 'I don't seem to be able to meet Mr Right. [My friend] says that all we need is a man . . . I don't think there's a Mr Right for people with mencaps.'[1]

This may change little by little as people with learning difficulties lead less sheltered lives and normalization progresses. People with a mental handicap who do marry seem to need less professional care as a couple than they did as single people.

Obviously the ability to marry depends on the ability to understand the nature of this commitment. Probably this is best learned by close friendship with an ordinary married couple who agree to befriend them over a fairly long period of time. What is important is to realize that marriage is not impossible for all people with mental handicaps.

McCarthy and Fegan[2] suggest that marriages planned by parents are not as likely to succeed as marriages planned by the couple themselves, who will then seek an advocate to help them fulfil their goal. Whether they marry or not, a couple with mental handicaps who have a sexual relationship will need contraceptive advice if nobody can be found to help them on a long-term basis with the care of consequent children.

Sterilization

The recent case of Jeanette, a seventeen-year-old girl in the care of Sunderland County Council whose mother wanted her daughter to be sterilized, illustrates the intensity of feeling aroused by such dilemmas. Considerable public concern from mental health agencies followed the High Court decision to permit sterilization before Jeanette reached the age of eighteen. An appeal to the Law Lords endorsed the High Court decision. The Secretary-General of Mencap expressed the widely held view that the decision would lead to more sterilization of girls with mental handicaps and to more restrictive patterns of care.

Lord Hailsham in announcing the decision said that it was made in her own interests. Moral, social and genetic issues were not relevant. Jeanette did not desire children, nor would she be able to look after a child. Her welfare was paramount and pregnancy would be an unmitigated disaster. The right to have a child is dependent on reproduction being the result of informed choices which Jeanette—the Law Lords said—could not make. The present legal position is that no one can give consent for a person with mental handicaps over the age of eighteen to be sterilized if they cannot give consent for themselves.[3]

One of the five Law Lords who made the decision was interviewed afterwards and said that any teenager under the age of 18 for whom sterilization is being considered should be made a ward of court. Each individual case should then be considered on its own merits in the High Court. A previous judgement seven years earlier which did not permit sterilization of an eleven-year-old girl was made by one of the few mothers who is a High Court Judge.

This case of Jeanette certainly exemplifies a difficult ethical decision. The ability to have children is valued by most women in our society. Permanently to remove it from a young woman because she has mental handicaps is a serious matter.

We do not know if Jeanette was consistently offered any teaching to help her discriminate degrees of social distance and to learn the behaviour appropriate to each, in the way we describe near the end of the previous chapter. Yet as a result of such teaching some women with learning difficulties are managing to avoid sexual exploitation and the consequent risk of unwanted pregnancy. Generally speaking it seems to us that, unless a sustained effort has been made over several years to teach appropriate social and sexual behaviour to an adolescent girl and until it becomes quite clear that she is not capable of such learning, it is selling her short to talk of her being permanently sterilized.

However, given that such teaching is not generally offered, we still have the problem of what to do with those who have not learned social skills and appropriate distancing. This will obtain until there is a more radical approach to sexual and relationship education as advocated here.

What about children?

Women with Down's syndrome have a 50 per cent chance of producing an affected child. Men with the complete Down's syndrome can have erections and ejaculate, but have not been known to father a child. However a few men with only a proportion of cells with the extra chromosome have fathered children. Apart from those with Turner's and Klinefelter's syndromes, most other people with learning difficulties are as likely to be as fertile as other people. Until now their lifestyle has made it less likely that they will become parents, but this could change in future.

Obviously parents with mental handicaps need a lot of education to appreciate the needs of children and to be able to meet them. One mother said:

> My handicapped daughter at sixteen talked endlessly about babies. She would have loved a baby, and for many years she played games that she had a baby of her own. When her younger sister married and had a baby they stayed with us at home. Suddenly she discovered that babies howl and scream and wet all over your lap. You have to change their nappies and feed them in the middle of the night. Since then she has gone right off babies and for the last ten years maintains that she would never like to have a baby.

Homosexual relationships

At the end of the last century and the early part of the twentieth century the Eugenic Society was active in promoting the growth of asylums outside our major cities. Segregation of the sexes was considered the only way to prevent heterosexual relationships, and thus reproduction. This extreme fear of reproduction was based on faulty ideas about genetics and on Morel's doctrine of degeneration, which held that if there was neurosis in one generation there would be psychosis in the second generation and retardation in the third. In fact, the children of people with a mental handicap will tend to be more intelligent than their parents.

We thus inherit a tradition of restricting people with mental handicaps to living exclusively with those of their own sex while depriving them of the company of the other sex. This can only encourage same-sex relationships and discourage heterosexual ones, and it seems likely that many who go on to adopt homosexual practices would in other circumstances have developed heterosexually.

Same-sex friendships are important for everybody, but especially for those deprived of heterosexual company. Friendships give a sense of being accepted, understood, valued and worthy, and they are to be fostered and encouraged. Homosexual genital acts are sometimes disregarded by care staff because 'at least there is no chance of pregnancy'. But, as with casual heterosexual intercourse, there is always the likelihood of exploitation, of disillusion, of a sense of bewilderment and a lowering of self-esteem. In this, as in other areas of living, care staff have a general responsibility to prevent the exploitation or damaging of one resident by another, and to do their best to remedy such damage as may inadvertently occur.

The Sexual Offences Act 1967 legalizes homosexual acts in private between no more than two consenting adult men over the age of 21. A person with a severe mental handicap cannot give his consent. However, it has been argued that two men, both of whom have severe mental handicaps, would not be in breach of the law by engaging in homosexual activity because neither could be expected to recognize the degree of impairment of his partner. There is no comparable legislation restricting homosexual acts between women.

The position of residential staff caring for sexually active men has not been clarified legally. Their best policy is to have 'decent intent' and consistently to follow guidelines discussed and agreed by all care staff together. Parents and pastoral care workers are entitled to ask residential staff what guidelines they have adopted with regard to sexuality.

It is not possible to deny the reality of adult sexuality, nor for staff to be blind to sexual activity when the only possibility for its expression is in open shared dormitories and bathrooms. Ideally sex education will emphasize the right to say 'No'. Ideally it will be offered to people who are allowed to choose friends of either sex. Ideally people with mental handicaps will live in small, friendly units with plenty of fulfilling occupations and minimal need for compulsive or obsessive sexual rituals. Certainly small group homes where men and women live together as a community seem more likely than large, single-sex institutions to offer the opportunity for satisfying heterosexual friendships.

Feeling, thinking and doing

Parents and care staff have many dilemmas in progressively helping people with learning difficulties to realize their sexual potential. This is often precisely because they must look openly and make sober judgements about situations which others directing their own sexual lives usually keep hidden or decide on impulse. One way for pastoral care workers to help parents and care staff with these dilemmas is to adapt an exercise from the Family Planning Association's book *Options for Change*[4] and to ask them to identify three factors. The first is how they *feel* about their son's masturbating or their resident's sharing bedrooms or cross-dressing, or whatever is the problem. The second is what they *think*, which will include what they know of good practice or ethical and religious principles or their understanding of the people concerned. The third is what is possible or what they would like to *do*, in the light of their thoughts and feelings.

Handle with care

Normalization implies that people with mental handicaps will exercise the greatest degree of choice that is possible for them. This means helping them to see what such choices involve. During a 'homelife' course residents in one small group home were consulted about the standards which would prevail in that home:

> Life is made up of choices, saying 'Yes' or 'No'. (Each resident looked in a full-length mirror and described which clothes he or she had said 'Yes' to that morning.) These are the little 'yes's'. The bigger 'yes's', like having sex with somebody or marrying, need preparation and care so as not to hurt ourselves and others. We have all been hurt in the past, so we must be extra careful. (A fine china coffee set with one broken cup was passed with infinite care from person to person to show how fragile things must be handled.) Residents then argued, agreed and dictated the house rules which they would observe to see that nobody got hurt. These included rules about answering the door, smoking and privacy.

Pastoral workers can help parents and carers to see that some degree of choice is always possible and encourage them progressively to increase that area of choice.

Summary

Loving relationships can be of great benefit to people with learning difficulties but sexual relationships without love may be damaging. Marriage and even child-bearing are not impossible, but they are likely to need most careful preparation and long-term support if they are to be successful. Same-sex friendships can be rewarding but sexual exploitation is to be avoided. The aim for carers is to help people with mental handicaps progressively to make their own sexual choices, to accept their responsibilities and to respect the rights of others.

Notes

1. Margaret Flynn and Christina Knussen, 'What It Means to be Labelled "Mentally handicapped" ' (*Social Work Today,* 16 June 1986).
2. Wendy McCarthy and Lydia Fegan, *Sex Education and the*

Intellectually Handicapped: a Guide for Parents and Care Givers.
ADIS Press (404 Sydney Road, Balgowlah, NSW 2093, Australia)
1984.

3. M. J. Gunn, 'Sex—the Present Law' (*Mental Handicap* 12, 3, 1984),
    pp. 104—6; 'Proposed Reform of Sexual Offences Legislation'(*Mental
    Handicap* 13, 1, 1985), pp. 16—37; 'Marriage' (*Mental Handicap* 14,
    1, 1986), pp. 37—8.

4. Hilary Dixon, *Options for Change*—Staff training handbook on
    personal relationships and sexuality for people with a mental handicap.
    Family Planning Association 1986.

SIX

All People Gathered

Before the Christian Church does anything, it must be church. It must be an assembly, a gathered people. And that means all people, rich and poor, old and young, male and female, black and white, healthy and sick, able and disabled. Part of the Church's richness is the diversity of people whom it gathers together. People with mental handicaps form part of the Church and supply some of that richness. Here is a picture of the impact made on one person by some of his fellow-parishioners:[1]

> I look forward now to Jamie greeting me with the thumbs-up sign as I come into church. Annie runs up and down during the service, and I catch her joy at being there. Sandy rocks backwards and forwards and crows at the solemn parts, while Robert bows low every time the priest does and copies his acts of blessing.
>
> Sandy goes to communion, and that has made a great impression on me. I used to be rather scrupulous about receiving communion: was I worthy, was I sufficiently recollected, did I pray as I ought? Then I saw Sandy at the altar rails and realized none of this matters, that to God we're all like Sandy. It is enough that we're present, that we want to share in this gift.

This account is remarkable because it describes people with severe learning difficulties who feel completely at home and accepted in their parish church and who are valued for their contribution there. How does this come about?

> It is hard to make a congregation aware so that they can all be welcoming, but we have found you can make some of the congregation very much aware. If you work with a few people they can become a sort of catalyst, the yeast in the leaven if you like, to teach the congregation as a whole. It is

really the welcome of the priest or the minister that is crucial and that is going to shape the attitudes of other people. If he or she can give the lead then all sorts of wonderful things can happen.

Frances Young, an ordained Methodist minister, describes the impact of her son Arthur upon one Easter congregation:[2]

> He joined the church breakfast, and Mrs Pemberton sat next to him. It was as though his presence liberated her, and she was able to take the lead in integrating him into the church family. To my delight and surprise one member of the congregation pushed him up to the communion rail so that he too shared the blessing of the children. It was a moving moment when I layed my hand on his head — and not just for me. Arthur was part of my ministry that weekend.

The church community starts to care

Pastoral care of people with severe learning difficulties begins at the moment parents are told that 'something is wrong':

> Pastoral care at this stage calls for compassion of the purest kind. There is little to say, but more can be done. The priest or parish worker who can take the baby in their arms, holding him or her warmly and lovingly, is speaking a thousand words. To sit with the parents and cry with them is sufficient. You know that that baby, made in the image and likeness of God, has a mission in the Church and in society and a role to play far exceeding the value our world may put upon her, upon him, but parents are scarcely ready for that yet. What they need is a presence which says, 'I am with you,' without words.

This is the time for pastoral workers to check whether parents are in touch with others who have been in the same situation, and to arrange this if they would like it. It is also the time for church people to start picking up any blank cheque they may have written earlier in the pregnancy:

> Today a new situation has arisen. The pregnant mother frequently undergoes pre-natal screening which may

indicate that the baby in the womb has some form of impairment or disability. An abortion may be proposed or even recommended.

What guidance can be given in this situation? Could you say, 'If your baby comes to term and is born handicapped the Church will be there'? There is a grave responsibility involved in making such a remark, but it pinpoints a crucial response to this dramatic situation. No church can campaign against abortion without living out the serious consequences of such a stand.

Accepting and naming a church member

The celebration of baptism can be immensely important to parents who may be feeling uncertain of society's attitude to their handicapped child:

> The priest, carefully using the child's name, needs to say that in the body of Christ every member has a role to play and that the child brings a gift which may only become clear later on in life. In holding the baby the priest, the representative of Christ in a special sense, speaks a powerful non-verbal message.

The baptism ceremony is also important for brothers and sisters:

> Too often the brothers and sisters are overlooked in the distress and drama surrounding the birth of a baby with a handicap. The baptismal ceremony provides them with recognition and an active supportive role which will hopefully establish their future position as equal members of the same family.

Where the baptism is performed during public worship the community has a chance to welcome the new parishioner and to offer support in many practical ways:[3]

> Small details like taking photos of the baby and family can mean much to the parents, some of whom are not yet ready to record the distinguishing features of handicap, yet in later years regret the gap in the family album. Indeed, it is especially important to children whose memory may be

limited or who may go eventually to residential care, that they have a pictorial record of their important life events.

Many House Church fellowships, Baptists, Pentecostals, Brethren and others offer believer's baptism by immersion.[4] The stunning symbolism of 'dying and rising' can be a profound gesture of incorporation into the body of Christ. The impact of total immersion in a large pool — the experience of wetness and washing — can be of great value to someone whose belief and understanding arises from their emotional intelligence rather than their cognitive intelligence.

Belonging and sharing

From the time of baptism children with mental handicaps are full members of the church community. When he is ready, when she is ready, they can be prepared for communion, the bread of life, but first they can experience giving and receiving the bread of friendship. Pastoral care is not solely the responsibility of the priest, and lay people can be involved in many different ways, babysitting, befriending parents and child, sharing outings and offering respite care, making friends too with brothers and sisters and seeing that they are not overshadowed in the general concern for the child with handicaps. Some parishes see the offering of friendship to families with a mentally handicapped child as too important to be left to chance, and nominate and prepare particular parishioners for this ministry.

A child with mental handicaps who has shared the bread of friendship in this way is soon ready to receive the bread of life.[5] One young man judged his readiness for himself:

Many Sundays passed of holding Nigel back at communion and trying to explain that he was not old enough — he was seven but could not put two words together. He knew he was 'like' other children in size though, and he had a natural respect for God. One Sunday everything seemed right for him to come to communion with me. We positioned ourselves at one end of the altar rails, and the priest paused to ask, 'Has he made his First Communion? 'No Father, this is it,' was my anxious reply! The only thing missing was the opportunity for a celebration with lots of other children, but that seemed a minor sacrifice for Nigel's new sense of belonging.

Choosing for oneself to belong

A person's full membership of the Church is celebrated at confirmation. Stephanie Clifford has long experience of preparing people with severe learning difficulties for this confirmation, and she distinguishes five principles:[6]

1. People who are mentally handicapped need a small group of believing adults, willing to build a welcoming and supportive community in which they can be prepared to receive the spirit of Jesus in confirmation.

2. Through baptism we belong to the Church, but this idea can so easily remain notional and abstract, and the small community of believing people makes sense of belonging, makes belonging real and concrete, and such a supportive group provides the contact for our people to agree to belong. And we know when they agree to belong, they will show us.

3. Membership of the Church implies a decision, the decision to belong to this small faith community. Being united to the church community or the parish may be the most concrete way that a person with a mental handicap can really identify with the Church. It may be the only church that he will ever know or ever understand, his little community. Then it is the bishop who affirms this commitment, and he confirms that person in the presence of the total church community. Through the sacrament of confirmation the bishop says to the person, 'Yes, you belong to the people of God.'

4. The bishop, if he is to be significant in forming this sense of belonging, must be seen as a friend rather than as a stranger. This funny man who appears out of the blue, dressed in a funny way: he has to be seen as a friend and therefore it is important that our people know him as a friend. The people I prepare for sacraments not only know him, they have tea with the bishop. It is important

that they eat with the bishop, but not only that; they prepare his crozier and polish up all his regalia ready for the confirmation ceremony so that they can identify with it, so that they can say, 'Oh look at that. How clean it is. I got it ready. I helped the bishop get ready.'

5. We are confirmed in the Spirit to exercise a ministry within our local church. That is for everybody, not just for some of us. Then as Christians we need to discover ways of allowing our people who are disabled in any way to exercise a ministry. There are many ministries open to people who are mentally handicapped, if we only just think. How wonderful they are at welcoming. They not only say 'Hello!' and welcome you, they lead you the whole way up the church and make sure you are comfortably installed. Serving, how they serve! Caring for vessels with pride: it is not a menial task, it is done with such pride. I know one young woman who could not find anything else to do so she started planting flowers in the priest's garden, and there was this beautiful patch of flowers which was used to enhance the altar. Also their greatest ministry, is it not the ministry of reconciliation? Is it not breaking down barriers that is their greatest apostolate, which must be recognized and named and spoken? Somehow I feel we should commission them to go out and break down barriers, and confirmation is the moment when we really do it.

Something to give

Whether or not they are confirmed members of the Church, people with severe learning difficulties can be involved in parish life much more than is often the case:

Looking positively and creatively for opportunities for integration will seldom be ineffectual. Serving on the altar, assisting the ushers, singing in the choir, joining the youth club or other activities for young people have all been successfully undertaken by people with mental handicap. Involvement may call for extra thought and maybe a friendly companion to walk alongside. It may require preparation so that others involved in the activity are welcoming and supportive.

Pastoral workers will recognize here the principle of normalization rightly understood: people with mental handicaps are not left to sink or swim, or expected to fight their own way into a parish, but the parish community is encouraged to look upon them as assets, as people with something to contribute, and actively to seek ways of helping them to make that contribution.

Should we hold special services?

The quest for a more ordinary life and for a place at ordinary pursuits has put a question mark over the holding of special services for people with mental handicaps.[7] Their inclusion into general church activities and worship as individuals in their own right is crucial and should not be compromised. Gathering people with learning difficulties into large groups and in some way singling them out as a special category seems in the main a retrograde step, both for their perception of themselves and for the attitudes of other worshippers towards them.

Yet there is a good case for sometimes holding public services which are not highly verbal and abstract, where Christians approach God and each other directly through song and mime, through gesture and touch, through music and atmosphere, through simple words deeply felt, through story and through symbol. If such occasional celebrations are carefully prepared and enacted, people with mental handicaps can take starring roles, but many others—including the young, the weary, the jaded and the intellectually punch-drunk—can discover release and refreshment themselves. The various Christian churches now have considerable experience of devising such celebrations, and these can form a collective contribution from people with mental handicaps and their families to other worshippers.

The other occasion when a special service seems entirely justifiable is when people with mental handicaps and their families are minded to gather in large numbers for a rally or jamboree. Many special-interest groups feel this need: to establish a sense of solidarity, to draw courage from each other, to give thanks for past achievements, to find strength for battles ahead, to create the euphoria which will sustain them through grey and lonely days awaiting them. Not even devotion to the principle of normalization need deprive people with mental handicaps or their families of a mass pilgrimage or a cathedral assembly of their very own.

A way to preach

The art of preaching well is rare. The art of preaching well to people with mental handicaps is surely rarer. To preach to a mixed congregation where some people have learning difficulties while others do not seems almost impossible. This chapter therefore concludes with the following sermon preached by Father David Wilson at the 1986 Mencap Service televised by the BBC.

A friend of mine was travelling home one evening on the underground. There were lots of people on the train. A young man was standing next to her. He gave her a big smile and said in a loud voice: 'It's my birthday today. I'm thirty-seven.' He told her what he'd been doing, and that there was going to be a party in the evening. They chatted away together for a few moments. When my friend got off at her station, another lady who had heard them talking said: 'Tsst tsst! Isn't it terrible—and he spoke in such a loud voice.' So my friend said: 'I wonder who was the more handicapped on the train. That young man or the rest of us with our long gloomy faces?'

The young man was someone we often call 'mentally handicapped.' There are those of you here and watching at home who are often labelled like this. Sometimes we think you won't notice, but from conversations I've had I know you do, and I know you don't like being labelled in that way. Sometimes we talk about you as if you weren't there and couldn't understand, but I know you do realize what's being said, and that you feel hurt when people speak *at* you, and not *to* you, and when you are left out of things. It's not nice to feel useless and different, as I know some of you have been made to feel. I want to say, 'Sorry,' to you for all the times I've shared in that.

We believe as followers of Jesus that everyone is important, that everyone has something to give. We believe that happiness, peace and joy come from hearts filled with love and God's Holy Spirit. They don't come from being specially clever at reading and writing and working things out or having a lot of money or a big job. Some people have these things but they feel empty inside, unhappy and unfriendly and often filled with fear.

We are not afraid to be ourselves; when we feel free to share our joys and sorrows; when we can say, 'Sorry', 'Welcome', 'Hello', and really mean it; when we can say with all our hearts, 'Jesus is my friend', then we are someone important. We need people like that here in London, in the cities, towns and villages all over the country.

I've gained so much from some of you, from Dorothy, Peter, Simon, Pius and from many others I include among my friends. I'm really grateful to you all. Thank you.

Summary

The Christian Church is an assembly, a people gathered together, and by definition includes in that gathering those people who have learning difficulties. They can feel at home in the Church and can make their own contribution to parish life.

As Terry Thompson, vice-chair of the newly formed Church Action on Disability says, 'We are saying to the Church: caring is not enough; acceptance is not enough. Disabled people are part of our congregation and it involves all of us.'

The priest or minister and other parish workers can be with parents as they learn of their child's disability and can offer practical help and friendship then and later. A person with mental handicaps can be prepared for and receive the Church's sacraments, and can be helped to find a place in the Church's regular work and worship. As long as individual integration is the norm, there is a place for occasional special services and sermons.

Notes

1. P. Gilbert, J. Healey, J. Hull, M. Rooney and B. Wycliffe, *We Are One People*. Diocese of Arundel and Brighton 1987.
2. Frances Young, *Face to Face*. Epworth Press 1985.
3. Pat Vassalo in David Wilson (ed.), *All People*. St Joseph's Centre (The Burroughs, Hendon, London NW4 4TY).
4. Faith Barnes (ed.), *Let Love be Genuine — Mental Handicaps and the Church*. Baptist Publications (Baptist Church House, Southampton Row, London WC1B 4AB) 1986.
5. Stephanie Clifford, *Invitation to Communion*. Kevin Mayhew 1980.
6. Stephanie Clifford, *Called to Belong: Preparing the Mentally Handicapped Person for Confirmation*. Kevin Mayhew 1984.
7. Stephanie Clifford, St Joseph's Mass Book. Collins 1985.

Further reading: Bryan George, *The Almond Tree*. Collins 1987.

SEVEN

Telling Sad Things

During a lifetime an individual experiences many losses. Some are losses of familiar relationships, experiences and places which are more or less planned. For example, moving house or changing school both involve the loss of well-known routines and people, and require the learning of new routines and getting to know new people. Coping with such losses and the associated changes in lifestyle is something we all have to learn to do.

Sometimes the loss causes a great deal of personal sadness. Nothing can adequately prepare us for the death of a close relative or friend. It is not possible to generalize about the importance of any particular loss. Its personal meaning will depend on the relationship which existed with the lost person and probably on earlier more or less satisfactorily resolved experiences of loss.

If a person with a mental handicap has consistently been protected from change, for example by maintaining the same routines, even a minor change in the caring arrangements may be very unsettling. Pastoral care workers will be familiar with statements describing such an individual — 'He doesn't like change', about day-to-day, minute-to-minute routines and rituals. Also familiar may be the assertion that 'he won't notice' when a relatively major change takes place, such as an elder sister leaving home to get married. The assumption seems to be that a person with learning difficulties is so wrapped up in his own world, that only things which directly impinge on his daily routine will be noticed.

A boarding school for children with learning difficulties was undergoing a major change of staff. The religious order which had founded the school were no longer able to staff it. Handing over to an entirely lay staff not only involved changes in the key positions of principal, matron and a member of the teaching staff, but required an increase in staff numbers to replace the out-of-hours cover they had also provided.

At the same time other members of the lay staff were leaving and the usual reorganization of classes and dormitories took place. At the start of the autumn term the changes which affected one pupil included a new teacher, new principal, new matron (whom he had to see daily for medication and exercises), new member of the care staff, new boys in his school class and new boys in his house (care) group. All in all seven key people in his life had left the previous term. Those who had left thought it best not to visit—perhaps thinking that they would cramp the style of the newcomers or that coming back to visit would remind those left behind of what they had lost. Coming back would have meant facing up to the pain of separation, facing up to questions spoken and not spoken:

'Did you go because you don't care any more?'

'Were we too naughty?'

'Have you forgotten us already?'

'Are you all right?'

Perhaps the new staff were aware of their own feelings of inadequacy as they attempted to replace people who were so highly regarded, and who had given so much. Whatever the reasons, when the children in the school were unsettled, homesick or even disturbed, the possibility that their recent experience of loss might be responsible was not considered.

The adjustment of this community to the changes which had taken place needed to be acknowledged, and the painful feelings of loss to be accepted.

The finality of death

There are three features of death which distinguish it from many other losses. The first is its irreversibility. The fact that someone will not breathe, nor eat, walk, talk or love ever again is a difficult and painful concept to grasp. Young children begin to understand this round about 5 or 6 years of age. They can be helped to understand the human life-cycle by learning about the rhythms of the natural world, and the life-cycle of other living things.

Take a goldfish, perhaps a child's treasured prize from the fair; its death will be sad but provides an ideal opportunity for learning. How many adults have disposed of the fish before the children notice? Do they say the fish died and leave it at that? Do they replace it with another? Do they talk about death and its finality? Children's literature is full of early death education. The first lullaby a mother sings to her child introduces the possibility of being abandoned:

> Rock-a-bye baby, on the tree top,
> When the wind blows, the cradle will rock,
> When the bough breaks, the cradle will fall,
> Down will come baby, cradle and all.

Of course a song like this is sung gently to a child and offers a chance to look at the realities of separation and loss from the safety of mother's arms. There are many other examples, including the nursery rhyme 'Humpty Dumpty' and the fairy stories 'Little Red Riding Hood' and 'Hansel and Gretel'.

The second feature which takes longer for children to understand is that every death is inevitable. The goldfish will die sooner or later. Within the experience of a small child a pet provides a manageable experience of both the finality and inevitability of death.[1]

It is much later that the universality of death is understood. Children are normally expected to achieve this by about the age of 9 or 10. Children and adults who have severe learning difficulties have been shown to take longer to understand these three rather abstract concepts. Perhaps one reason for this delay is the difficulty their parents and carers have in explaining and sharing experiences of death.

Dependent relationships and loss

The most important feature which distinguishes those people who have a mental handicap from those who don't is the dependence of the former on their parents. The inevitability of their own death causes some parents to harbour death wishes for their children, and others to experience feelings of relief if their child does die before them. In the normal run of things their child with a mental handicap will still be dependent when they themselves die. The major task of parenthood is to enable children to become fully independent. This is an aim which can at best be only partially fulfilled for a child with long-lasting dependency needs.

Parents react to this dilemma in different ways. Sometimes they accept the dependency totally and discourage any moves towards separation — apparently denying the reality of their own limited life-expectancy. Sometimes they reject their child, feeling that the demands to care are excessive and beyond the limits of their own personal resources. Most tread an uncertain path between meeting dependency needs and offering frequent, carefully planned experiences of separation; between accepting the ultimate responsibility for their child and learning to share this responsibility with the wider community; between making decisions for their child and encouraging him to make even the simplest choices for himself.

Facing the possibility that their child will live for twenty or thirty years after their own death pushes other parents into making detailed arrangements for their child's care for the rest of his life. For example they may have taken professional advice in drawing up their wills, and may have set up a family trust or left a legacy to Mencap. They may have arranged with Mencap to provide a lifelong visiting service through their Trustee Visitors Scheme, in the way described by Gerald Sanctuary.[2]

Letting go

Pastoral workers can gently encourage parents to make such practical arrangements. Yet, although such preparations may help, it is not always enough to 'do' things to make the way ahead easier. A death wish on the part of the parent can be a powerful generator of guilt and of murderous fantasies. Two mothers attending a parents' group which was focusing on the difficulties of letting go their adult children shared their uncomfortable feelings about this. They both admitted to keeping a small stock of sleeping pills with the intention of overdosing their dependent child when they knew their own death was imminent. Completing practical arrangements may afford parents considerable peace of mind, perhaps by discharging some of their guilt. Just as importantly, it can prepare them emotionally for the final separation. Parents are less likely to blame themselves for letting go of their adult sons and daughters with mental handicaps if pastoral workers help them to face up to the fact that such separation is normal for other young adults. Letting go of one's adult children usually happens in the late teens or early twenties. There are good reasons for looking for new lives, away from parents, for young adults with learning difficulties at the same age. Parents are ready to move into a different stage of their own lives when parenting is complete. Opportunities for new leisure interests can be explored before retirement from regular work occurs. Changing responsibilities within a marriage, as well as for single parents, provoke changes in relationships with adult sons and daughters too.

Yet for some parents dedicated to caring for their adult sons and daughters such considerations may seem almost selfish.

A group of parents of young adults with mental handicap were discussing their emotional difficulty in making arrangements for their sons and daughters to leave home. Caring for their child had been 'a struggle at first,' said one mother, 'but we finally switched ourselves on to taking responsibility for her twenty-four hours a day, seven days a week. Will somebody now please tell us how to switch ourselves off?' Others agreed that alongside them as they shouldered responsibility for their child went the fear, 'What will happen when I'm gone?' This fear was never faced squarely, but was met by steadfastly renewing their resolution to cope as long as possible. 'How can we give up now?'

The counsellors working with these parents obtained a filmed extract showing part of the Cardiff NIMROD scheme,[3] in which a social worker was teaching a middle-aged man with Down's syndrome the living skills which might enable him to return and care for himself in his family home, which he had been forced to leave upon his widowed father's death.

The man (called Jimmy) described this death and spoke movingly of his love for his father. Yet parents watching could see that, for all his care, the father had left his son unable to use money, or shop, or cope with traffic, or to eat out, all of which he proved capable of learning. If the beloved father had also managed to teach these skills, Jimmy need never have experienced the upset of having to leave home after he died. 'I see now that my task is to work myself out of a job in my lifetime,' concluded one mother, 'Not to soldier on till I drop.'

For the individual who is disabled in some way, a gradual transition from dependence on parents to a lifestyle which is separate will be easier to achieve while parents are able to encourage and approve. Regular visits to their child's new home, and by their adult child to the parental home will help the separation to succeed. It is essential however that the individual's emotional ties continue to be respected.

One young man had settled well into a home which he shared with a few other people. When his father died he was not informed immediately. It was not the fault of the hospice, but the family did not tell him until the funeral was over. A week later he went out and vandalized some cars in the area. He was admitted to hospital for long-term care and lost his place in the group home. There was no recognition of his grief.

Derek was thirty-two and had always lived at home with his parents who were now in their seventies. He was an only child, and had Down's syndrome. Derek attended a day centre, but since his father retired had been irregular in his time-keeping and had chosen to stay at home once or twice weekly. He had been on holiday with the centre, but preferred family holidays. He was admitted to hospital immediately after his last summer holiday, with a high temperature and complaining of a sore throat and abdominal pain. He stopped eating and drinking, and did not speak for several days. When he resumed talking, it was in a whisper. Concern about his deteriorating physical health resulted in extensive investigations, and Derek was fed through a nasogastric tube. Later he was fed intravenously.

Some months later when the clinical situation had deteriorated even further, a second psychiatric opinion was sought. A careful review of his recent life history revealed the death of his mother's sister some months earlier of stomach cancer. Another significant piece of information was that the aunt always used to holiday with Derek and his parents, and her symptoms were similar to his and began on their shared holiday a year earlier. Derek had shown no signs of grief at the time of her death although he had been very fond of her.

It was apparent that he did not have an adequate understanding of the ageing process, nor of the normal life-cycle, and had not understood the permanence of his aunt's death. The holiday experience probably precipitated a delayed grief reaction.

It was surmised that Derek had begun to recognize his parents' mortality since his aunt's death, and had decided to die first.

In such a serious situation very skilled help is needed to help the individual towards a planned separation in his parents' lifetime. Only then will he be able to find a new interest in living through relationships and activities which do not involve his parents.

The dying person

Just as the need to grieve for other people's deaths is often overlooked, so is the need for people with mental handicaps to prepare for their own death. The head teacher of a special boarding school reacted to the teaching video *The Last Taboo: Mental Handicap and Death*[4] with the comment that death was fortunately not a common part of their school life. Sadly a few weeks later an eighteen-year-old pupil was diagnosed as having a terminal illness. Edward had many questions about his illness. Will I get better? Does it hurt to die? Why is Mummy crying?

Accompanying someone in the last few days and hours of their journey on earth brings the possibility of one's own death nearer too. The task includes helping the dying person to let go of worldly possessions and of friendships, and to realize that his relationship with God is all important. Dying with dignity is possible with familiar people there to comfort you.[5]

Understanding grief

Grief following the death of a close relative or friend is a normal and common reaction. Bereavement counselling is available to many people through an individual's church, voluntary organizations such as CRUSE or through health and social service agencies. Someone who has a mental handicap may be just as much in need of counselling, but it is unusual for this help to be offered.

Pastoral workers or counsellors may have little experience of being with people who have learning difficulties. They may feel ill at ease, or inadequately skilled in communicating. They may have difficulty understanding the problems of the grieving person. For example in trying to respect the individual's need to know, how much information is appropriate? The enormity of the loss may affect pastoral workers themselves as they find the painful feelings too difficult to share. If the grieving person also has special problems such as a visual or hearing impairment or a physical disability, these problems may get in the way of the attempt to understand. Trying to understand and to explain and comfort are vital. Perhaps a genuine and sustained attempt to communicate and share will convey enough emotionally. An intellectual understanding of the permanence of a loss is less necessary. Our senses of sight and hearing and touch will reinforce our realization of our loss. The person is not there, the bed is empty, as is the place at table. At the funeral service the coffin and the flowers are seen and perhaps touched. The funeral music and singing is heard, as are the subdued voices of the mourners. Being a mourner and joining in the rituals of the funeral helps each one of us to come to terms with our loss.

Common human reactions

Grief has been described as a passive condition of helplessness, and mourning as the active reaction to grief.[6] The work of mourning acts to make real the fact of the loss. Thus attending the funeral, sorting out the clothes of the deceased person and other necessary tasks are helpful although painful reminders of the loss.

The emotional bonds to the deceased person must slowly be undone. Thus activities which were shared must now be done alone or with someone else. Tasks which were done on your behalf by the deceased person must now be done by yourself or by someone new. Finally readjustment to an environment from which the deceased person has irrevocably gone is necessary. If this also involves a change of environment because of your dependency, the readjustment may be prolonged.

The expression of grief has been well described by Kübler-Ross[7] and Parkes.[8] Feelings of shock, panic and denial are common early reactions which may give way to anger or guilt. Blaming oneself or someone else may help to diffuse and confuse the pain of the loss. Later the realization of the finality of the loss leads to feelings of depression and finally to acceptance and to reorganization of one's life without the dead person. Working through this bereavement response may take many months, and feelings of grief may recur months or years later at an anniversary or other reminder of the lost person.

Looking more closely, the following responses are described by people who have been bereaved; feelings of fear and panic, feelings of disbelief about what has happened, feelings of remorse, feeling out of control, being under or over-active, losing an appetite for food, being unable to sleep, having a poor memory, hearing the voice of the dead person, wanting to talk to them, forgetting they have died, being cross with other people, crying a lot, being unable to think or work.

Grief and mental handicap

For someone with a mental handicap the same reactions may be expressed behaviourally rather than through speech. Disturbances of sleep and appetite are relatively easy to notice. Denial of the death or a failure to understand its finality may lead to searching behaviour. Unexplained anger towards objects or people or episodes of self-injury may be harder to understand. A loss of intellect or other skills and the loss of bladder control may seem completely unrelated. Our difficulty is in recognizing behavioural manifestations of grief—especially if the apparent response to the death is one of indifference.

When thirteen-year-old Emma's grandad died, she went straight to her bedroom. Her mother thought she had not taken the news in. An hour later she heard a banging sound. Emma was kicking her bedroom door. Emma's mother didn't understand straightaway, but shouted to her 'to calm down'. Then she said to Emma, 'You're upset about Grandad!' Emma cried. Her Gran didn't want her to attend the funeral in case she was upset. But Emma enjoyed herself and in her somewhat uninhibited way helped the other mourners to talk about Grandad.

John was thirty-two years old. He had a severe mental handicap; he could not speak and understood very little spoken language. John had lived in a traditional institution for people with mental handicap for thirteen years since his mother died. His dependency needs were met by a dedicated team of nurses. His lifestyle was uneventful, most days being spent in the dayroom of his ward. Little attention was paid to his individuality, and none of the nurses knew his life history. One of the unqualified staff had known John since he was first admitted, but usually nurses only stayed for two or three years at the most. Recently John had been staying in bed and refusing to eat. He had been scratching his face, and the nurses were worried he might damage his eyes.

Careful attention to John's life history by the visiting psychiatrist reminded the staff that his father used to visit him weekly. The last record of him visiting was six months previously. A presumptive diagnosis of morbid grief with depression was made, and it was later confirmed that his father had died. John responded slowly to treatment with antidepressant medication. Grief counselling was not attempted, and the staff caring for John were reluctant to acknowledge his emotional needs.

Guidelines
Because of the difficulty in recognizing grief reactions in

people with mental handicap it may be helpful to suggest some guidelines. In fact the same guidelines relate to everyone—not just to people with severe learning difficulties.

It is not a good idea to change one's living arrangements soon after the death of a close relative. For someone with a mental handicap every effort should be made to help them to stay in their own home for as long as possible. The same advice is given to widows—decisions to move house should be deferred for at least six months. In the same way changes in daily activities should be approached cautiously, especially if any element of assessment or training is required. If an individual may have lost skills, he will need all his emotional energy to regain them—not to acquire new ones. It is not a good time for anyone to take on a new job.

These guidelines require that everyone involved in the care of the person with a mental handicap knows and understands about his bereavement. It follows that anticipatory training is needed to prepare carers for the possibility of an individual in their care being bereaved.

Sadly it is often the case that the death of a parent will be the start of a chain of losses. Admission to residential care may be inevitable, possibly some distance away from home, resulting in a change of daily activity and the loss of friends and familiar staff. The bereaved person may be worried about who is feeding the cats or bringing in the post—tasks which perhaps had been theirs for years. Even the milkman will be different. None of the old familiar routines will be experienced again, and it is not unknown for the family home to be disposed of without the handicapped individual ever going back. David Cook's novel, *Walter*, movingly describes this sad sequence of events.[9]

Bereavement counselling

The task here is to help with the work of mourning. There are practical ways in which someone can be helped to understand the finality of their loss, like joining in the funeral rituals, and experiencing the loss through seeing and hearing and touching. Helping someone to say goodbye may involve the counsellor in revisiting the grave or the home of the deceased person with the bereaved person and in looking at photographs or other mementoes with him or her. The bereaved person may need permission to express negative feelings about their dead relative; feelings about being let down or deserted. The counsellor is in a position to understand how normal such feelings are, whereas a carer may discourage an individual in her care from 'speaking ill of the dead'.

Maureen's mother died in her seventies. She had never been away from home, and did not settle well into hostel life with twenty-five other people. She repeated endlessly that all would be well if her mother came back. Helping Maureen required her to accept the loss of her mother before she could begin to make sense of her new life. She was able to revisit her old home and see that her mother no longer lived there. She visited her mother's grave and was able to express some anger. Later it was possible for her to think positively about her wish to live in an ordinary house in the community, sharing with some people her own age.

Summary

People with mental handicap need help to avoid the problems which may follow a bereavement. Maureen Oswin has drawn up some detailed recommendations for professionals:[10]

1. All professionals working with mentally handicapped people should inform themselves of normal grief reactions. They should make contact with local branches of CRUSE, the organization concerned for bereaved people.

2. Everyone coming into contact with bereaved mentally handicapped people should respect their right to be told the truth and to grieve.

3. Parents should try to have a plan of action in the event of deaths (for example, as in the Harrow Weald Mencap branch document). It could also be helpful if local branches of Mencap had links with local branches of CRUSE.

4. Day centre staff should have a plan of action in the event of a student becoming bereaved while at the centre.

5. Immediate removal to an unfamiliar residential facility should be avoided when a bereavement occurs. It would be kinder for the bereaved person to have a professional or volunteer or friend staying with them in their own home for the first two or three nights and then to move gradually into the residential facility.

6. Assessment should be avoided in the early months following a bereavement, because the mentally handicapped person may be functioning at a lower level of ability during this critical time.

7. Multiple residential care placements should be avoided.

8. Every attempt should be made to ensure continuity of staff in the residential facility, with an assigned member of the care staff wherever possible.

9. If the bereavement results in the person losing their home they should have a full explanation about what has happened to it and they must be permitted to take into residential care some belongings which are important to them.

Anticipation of loss is essential, and extra effort is needed to understand what any loss means to a handicapped person. The right to be told the truth and to be allowed to grieve must be respected.

Notes

1. Marlee and Benny Alex, *Grandpa and Me*. Lion 1981.
2. Gerald Sanctuary, *After I'm Gone — What Will Happen to My Handicapped Child?* Souvenir Press 1985.
3. *NIMROD — Mental Handicap in Wales*. Applied Research Unit, Ely Hospital, Cowbridge Road, Cardiff CR5 5XE.
   The NIMROD Story, a video. Available from Concord Video, 201 Felixstowe Road, Ipswich IP3 9BJ.
4. L. Sireling and S. Hollins, *The Last Taboo — Mental Handicap and Death*: A teaching video, 1985. Available from the Department of

Psychiatry, St George's Hospital Medical School, Cranmer Terrace, London SW17 0RE.

5. Sarah Boston, *Will, My Son — the Life and Death of a Mongol Child.* Pluto Press 1981.
6. B. Schoenberg *et al., Psychosocial Aspects of Terminal Care.* Columbia University Press, New York, 1972.
7. Elisabeth Kübler-Ross, *Living with Death and Dying.* Souvenir Press 1981.
8. C. Murray Parkes, *Bereavement — Studies of Grief in Adult Life.* Penguin 1986.
9. David Cook, *Walter*: Penguin 1980.
10. Maureen Oswin, (1985): 'Bereavement', in Craft, Bicknell and Hollins (ed.), *Mental Handicap.* Balliere Tindall 1985.

EIGHT

Who Cares Now?

Present-day patterns of care are paradoxical. To begin to understand them, pastoral workers need to look back in time at social and legal reform. The practices and laws of each age derived from prevailing views and prejudices. The range of erroneous beliefs held about someone with a mental handicap have varied from the fear that he or she was the devil's child to the hope that the person was holy and God-given. This chapter gives the background against which current struggles to provide suitable care are taking place.

A historical perspective

In the most primitive hunting and foraging societies the handicapped individual would have had difficulty surviving. As societies began to organize their resources, disadvantaged individuals began to expect to have a share. In England in 1325 the earliest recorded statute addressing the needs of the 'idiot' allowed for his property to be protected and profits from the land to be used for his benefit. No formal provision was made to support needy individuals, but they would remain members of their village communities. As people moved into the towns in increasing numbers, richer people contributed to the care of paupers and others through a system of parish relief. The Poor Law of 1601 led to the development of the workhouse where society's misfits could find shelter. People who were thought of as invalids, tramps, paupers, insane people and idiots all found asylum together in an increasing number of institutions which provided human warehousing if nothing else. Eventually in 1847 the first asylum specifically for people with mental handicap was built at Parkhouse in Highgate (in 1866 it moved to Surrey to become the Royal Earlswood), followed in 1870 by the

Darenth Training Schools. Also in 1886 the Idiocy Act set out the procedures for registration and for admission and discharge. At around the same time industrial development highlighted the need for education of the workers. Child labour was abolished and the 1870 Elementary Education Act made education more or less compulsory. It soon became apparent that some children could not master even the most basic literacy and numeracy skills. This led to a new law in 1899 empowering schools to ascertain which children were 'defective' and to make some provision for those who were considered educable. The Royal Commission on the Care and Control of the Feeble Minded reported in 1908. Pressures on them from the Eugenic Society were resisted, and they recommen 'ed that 'defectives' should be certified and segregated for their own protection and happiness, rather than to improve any genetic characteristics.

The 1913 Mental Deficiency Act introduced legal powers to admit and to detain handicapped people in hospital; a situation which remained virtually unchanged until the 1959 Mental Health Act, when people were enabled to enter and leave mental hospitals informally. The number of people in institutions rose steeply from about 5,000 at the beginning of the twentieth century to 70,000 in 1970. The Victorian-built institutions quickly became overcrowded, and men and women were segregated to avoid any risk of pregnancy.

The response of our modern human service agencies

The medical and nursing professions accepted increasing responsibility for different aspects of care for people with mental handicap. The 1944 Education Act had still deemed some children ineducable. The health authorities set up Junior Training Centres to provide day care for them. After the 1949 National Health Service Act even the task of providing somewhere to live for people with severe learning difficulties, formerly a local authority responsibility, was transferred to the health authorities.

Changing attitudes in the post-war period allowed the health authorities to do a fairly quick turn around. Having accepted the medicalization of the care provided for people with handicaps in the 1940s, by the late 1950s they were again asking local authorities to provide homes and day centres for them. In the event the response was slow and hospital admissions continued to rise. Throughout the 1960s scandals in many of these large institutions led to government reaction in the form of the 1971 White Paper, 'Better Services for the Mentally Handicapped'.[1] This paper described the inadequacies in current hospital and social service provision, and laid down norms for service developments in the next twenty years. Recommendations included running down the hospital population through an active policy of discharging people. Social services were asked to develop a range of residential and daycare facilities, to avoid inappropriate new admissions to hospital, and to welcome discharged people back into the community. Health and social service professionals were encouraged to work more closely together, and to develop a multi-disciplinary approach to assessing and providing for each person's needs. The National Development Team—a government watchdog of services—was formed under the chairmanship of Professor G. Simon at the Department of Health and Social Security. However a White Paper has no statutory power, and the services which have evolved during the 1970s and 1980s vary enormously in quality from one place to another. The hospital population has fallen by about one thousand a year but not primarily because of any successful discharge policy. The resident population of most institutions is an ageing one, and the reduction in numbers is partly because people who die are no longer replaced by new admissions.

New homes for old

Home life for children was improved dramatically by a new government policy in the early 1980s that no children under sixteen years old should live in hospital. Extra money was provided to move children into small homes in the community, and fostering and adoption agencies increased their expertise in placing severely handicapped children with families. For example, Dr Barnardo's Homes have been at the forefront of demonstrating new models of care for children who were formerly considered in need of medical and nursing care.

Respite care

Children with learning difficulties are children first. They have all the same needs as any child for love, security and for consistency. For parents who cannot cope with the constant demands of caring, a shared care arrangement may be created. Sometimes it has been too easy to forget that the same guidelines apply for these children as for others: in most cases it is not good practice to separate young children from their parents. Maureen Oswin has written graphically about the reality of short-term (respite) care provision in *They Keep Going Away* (see p. 27, n.2). It makes sobering reading.

Educational opportunities

Not until the 1970 Education Act were all children with mental handicap given the right to education. Children were classified as moderately or severely subnormal — terms which were changed by the most recent Education Act in 1981 to moderate or severe learning difficulty.

The story of Charnwood, an integrated nursery centre in Stockport, is described by Grace Wyatt.[2] She began pioneering work in the 1960s by inviting children with severe handicaps to attend every day with their normal peers. Such innovative projects paved the way for later development in statutory services.

Children with learning difficulties do need additional help. Many factors may conspire instead to reduce the choices actually available. Extra effort must be made to accept children with special educational needs into ordinary playgroups, nursery and primary schools. If a child needs extra help to make use of such opportunities, there is now a route through which this can be provided. The 1981 Education Act requires that all children with special educational needs will have a statement made of this need and the required educational support. It also recommends that wherever possible children will be educated in an ordinary school. So for example John, who has Down's syndrome, attends his local infant school and is the same age as the other children in his class. He joins all the children for games, music and art but has his own part-time teacher to set numeracy and literacy work at his own level.

The parent movement

Changes in attitudes since the Second World War have in large part been due to the growth of parent organizations. In 1946 Judy Fryd founded the Association of Parents of Backward Children, which is now the Royal Society for Mentally Handicapped Children and Adults (Mencap). In 1960 fifteen national parent organizations brought their shared concerns together to found the International League of Societies for Persons with Mental Handicap. There are now nearly a hundred affiliated societies worldwide. The League has international conferences and publications which help national organizations to influence their own governments. Parent groups were tremendously encouraged by the formation of the US President's Panel on Mental Retardation and its 1962 report. That the Kennedy family did not hide the fact of Rosemary Kennedy's mental handicap encouraged other families not to hide away their children. Parents, united by their children's needs, began to demand the best care that society could provide. Together they found strength to challenge traditional professional practices. They successfully fought for better state benefits, education and personal care. Much of their current energy is directed towards enabling integration into the community. They recognize that the social problems of everyday living are a bigger obstacle to achieving this than the provision of housing. Their major aim is to achieve the full acceptance of people with handicaps.

As with all movements, counter-movements spring up to challenge directions which seem too extreme to some. In the UK there is a relatively new parent organization called Rescare—the National Society for Mentally Handicapped People in Residential Care. This sees the care in the community initiative as a threat to their children's security. Most of the members are parents of adult children who are in hospital care, and who wish to retain for them the protection and stability that their present care affords. They are demanding the means to transform their hospital homes into segregated village communities.

The true burden of care in the community will fall on parents or other immediate carers' shoulders unless additional help is made available. The members of Rescare doubt whether such help will be provided, or worry that it will be vulnerable to political and economic expediency.

Pastoral care workers new to working with people who have mental handicaps may be forgiven for finding these divisions among parents confusing. On the same day they may meet one set of parents fully accepting the closure of a hospital and fighting for better care within the community and another set of parents doing battle to keep the hospital open and convinced that community care will mean no care at all. The happiest outcome would be to maximize real choice for parents and for their sons and daughters with mental handicaps. Some residential care would remain in homes and units with good staffing and standards of care. At the same time extra help would be forthcoming to make care in the community a reality. Equally, pastoral care workers will find among parents of school-age children the same kind of divisions. Many parents fight long and bitter battles to have their children accepted along with their neighbours' at the local mainstream school. Other parents campaign for the special schools to remain open and well resourced, fearing that their children will be submerged in the mainstream hurly-burly and their special needs remain unmet. The best outcome would be to work for good examples of both types of education. In that way parents may have the widest choice and children the chance of varied sorts of education to meet their different needs.

Current philosophies of care

There are many models of care world-wide based on the normalization principle which have shown that it is possible to base a service around individual needs in ordinary domestic environments. The King's Fund project paper *An Ordinary Life*[3] states:

> Our goal is to see mentally handicapped people in the mainstream of life, living in ordinary houses in ordinary streets, with the same range of choices as any citizen, and mixing as equals with the other and mostly not handicapped members of their own community.

The Committee of Enquiry into Mental Handicap Nursing

and Care (Jay Report 1979)[4] took serious note of such projects and concluded that people with mental handicap have a right to enjoy normal patterns of life in the community. They recommended some new principles of care which included:

A proper separation of home, work and recreation.
The opportunity to leave home in adulthood.
The choice of living in a mixed environment.
Additional help for individuals to achieve their potential.

Community-based services are struggling to keep pace with the demand.

In 1981 the government published a document called *Care in the Community* which suggested a number of mechanisms for transferring funds from health to social services. This transfer of money was expected to accelerate the development of community resources. However the availability of financial resources must be accompanied by changes in staff attitudes and by intensive staff training for the very different work of caring in the community. Building up a welcoming community is a slow process, bedevilled by rapid staff turnover and difficulties in staff recruitment. In the communities of the International Federation of L'Arche the emphasis is firmly on the formation of a welcoming community. Individuals with handicaps are then invited to live with people who are ready to care and to share their own lives, and who are supported by this wider community. Here too people's spiritual and emotional needs are given as high a priority as their physical and material needs.

Many pastoral care workers who read this book will have opportunities to extend their care so that it includes those people in their area who have learning difficulties. For example, it may be by befriending 'the new people at number 6', a group home for three adults. Professional help will have been provided but the friendly ear of someone with the time to listen is more difficult to programme. Or it may be as a priest or marriage-guidance or bereavement counsellor. Pastoral workers who are willing to include people with learning difficulties among their clients should think carefully if they are readily accessible to this group of people. Do they need to make known their willingness, perhaps by getting to know the specialist services in the locality?

'Living in the community' conjures up many different living situations. It may mean living with an exhausted family because there are no alternatives. Increasingly the choice available will include staffed and unstaffed group homes and flats, small hostels, warden-supported bedsitters, board and lodging, family living schemes offering both child and adult fostering and other options. Ann Shearer gives many examples of good practice in her book *Building Community*.[5]

Pastoral workers reflecting on the emphasis given to the new models of care might be forgiven for asking whether service designers give much thought to what people want. Surely choice is more important than exalting any particular good above others.

Day care

At the same time as there is a change in the philosophy of residential services towards a normalization model, day care services are undergoing major changes too. During the 1960s it was found that even people with severe mental handicaps could be taught to perform industrial assembly tasks at speed. Industrially-orientated Adult Training Centres accepted contracts for the assembly of light parts and components. This industrial emphasis meant that the continued education and social development of individual adults tended to be neglected. Fewer contracts are available now because of changes in the industrial economy, and thus a re-evaluation of the objectives of training centres has been forced. In many places Adult Training Centres were renamed Social Education Centres to reflect more accurately their social and educational programmes. Even this change, which was seen as so progressive a few years ago, is resented by some people who do not like to be seen as eternal students. In some centres staff and clients now call each other centre members. Where salaried work opportunities are provided, these are in both sheltered and integrated working environments. The Mencap Pathway Employment Scheme is one good example in which people are carefully introduced to work in the open market and supported and counselled by a special employment officer.

Are hospital facilities still needed?

Th˄ 1971 White Paper suggested that 27,000 hospital beds would still be needed by 1990. It is widely accepted that this was a gross overestimation. Views vary considerably about the practicality of enabling all people whatever their dependency needs to live more ordinary community-based lives. For example, some people believe that anybody showing disturbed behaviour should be cared for in hospital. An opposite view is that such people are best supported in their own home where problem behaviours are more likely to resolve. Some health authorities are developing specialist health care (in-patient) units for assessment and short-term treatment, or for long-term residential care for certain special groups. Examples of such groups are those with severe behaviour problems, people with additional sensory handicaps and those with multiple handicaps.

A more important development since the early 1970s has been the creation of various services to support families and people with mental handicap in their own homes.

Extra help

People with mental handicap and their carers need a network of support throughout their local community. They need to know where extra help can be found, and who will be able to advise them. Many local agencies produce a directory of information, such as the Wandsworth Directory, *Who Can Help*,[6] which is an A to Z of local resources for everything from A for Access to W for Word Blindness, or Mencap's *London Directory of Services*[7] for families and young children with special needs. The network will probably include early support and intervention schemes for newly diagnosed children, parent linking and befriending, sitting in and respite care, toy libraries and incontinence supplies, opportunity groups, day care and holiday play schemes, counselling and support groups, specialist health care, practical and financial help, fostering schemes and so on. All these schemes help to share the burden of care with each family.

Edna Wallace has promoted the idea of 'preview' (or preventive review)[8] as one of the best ways of letting carers of people with mental handicap know that their problems have been understood. This is a crisis prevention approach which relies on identifying certain critical stages in the life of an individual before they present as a crisis. Where preview is beginning to happen, families or individuals who are known to the computerized mental handicap register can be contacted at predetermined intervals to assess their needs.

Up to the age of about thirteen the professional contributions to care will be drawn from the paediatric services, from education and from social services. Now it is time for the Community Mental Handicap Team to become involved to help a smooth transition from children's to adult services. A critical time during a young adult's life is at the school-leaving age. The first preview will be convened by the social services department during the preceding year. The aim will be to highlight the child's future needs and to contribute to plans for education and specialist care. This is also an opportunity to remind parents about statutory benefits such as attendance and mobility allowances to which they may be entitled. In particular, note will be taken of additional handicaps such as epilepsy, physical disability or problem behaviours. Thereafter 5-yearly preview meetings are suggested so that carers know long-term help will be available in planning future care 'when we can no longer cope'. After the age of fifty more frequent preview may be appropriate. This approach requires a major commitment by social services departments and is not very widespread. The proponents hope that prevention will lead to a more efficient and humane use of resources.[9]

In the UK the local authority is responsible for providing a place to live for those who are homeless or who cannot provide their own home. It also has an obligation to provide daytime activities for adults in conjunction with the education department. The health authority is responsible for meeting everyone's health care needs, and increasingly people with mental handicap are using ordinary mainstream services. Some specialist health and social service resources are also needed; one example is the Community Mental Handicap Team.

One model of professional service provision — the Community Mental Handicap Team

The National Development Team has recommended that there should be one Community Mental Handicap Team for every 60 — 80,000 people. Every person with a mental handicap who lives within this geographic area, or who has been admitted to residential care elsewhere but previously lived within the area, is entitled to request help from the team.

The idea is to have a team based in the local community which will accept referrals from parents, people with mental handicap, doctors, social workers, and so on and will meet the specialist health care needs of people with mental handicap. A good team will develop to meet local needs so it is not possible to describe a typical team in detail.

The Community Mental Handicap Team is a multi-disciplinary team usually including community mental handicap nursing, psychiatry, clinical psychology and social work. Increasingly other skills available to people with mental handicap through the Community Mental Handicap Team include occupational, speech and physiotherapy, dietetics, family planning and health education.

By working together in a team and sharing knowledge across disciplines, it should be possible to enhance the service offered to each client. One person in the team will be nominated the 'keyworker' for each client to co-ordinate all contact with that client and his carers. The person chosen will be the one with the most relevant skills according to the nature of the request for help. In addition to their own professional role, and the keyworker role, team members are expected to provide a link to one or more agencies in the catchment area by regular contact. This might be a group home or a hostel, a day centre or a club. The link person's task is to provide an easy route for referrals to the team and an opportunity for information exchange. Team members are thus contributing to the development of a supportive network of care, and are more readily able to direct clients to other useful resources. Liaison with social services is an important component of the team's work.

The keyworker discusses the client's progress with the rest of the team and will invite other disciplines to make an assessment or contribute to developmental or treatment programmes as necessary. This process of drawing up a programme and writing the resulting plan down may be part of an Individual Programme Planning system.[10] At the heart of this system is the commitment to make decisions jointly between the client, his or her family and a small number of other people who have regular contact with him or her. Information is gathered before the planning meeting so that the time can be devoted to identifying needs and deciding goals and who will be responsible for each goal.

Jason is nineteen and lives at home with his widowed mother. Jason has had major fits since he was a young child. He went to a special school for children with moderate learning difficulties until he was sixteen. His mother approached the Community Mental Handicap Team when Jason was depressed because he could not get a job, and asked for help to get him out of the house a bit more. A community nurse became his keyworker and offered him regular supportive counselling, and introduced him to other opportunities in the borough. He has recently accepted a place in a Social Education Centre and is in the prework group. A psychiatric assessment resulted in Jason being offered a place in a psychotherapy group for young adults with learning difficulties to increase his understanding and acceptance of his disability. His mother joined a parents group which was focusing on the problems for parents of 'letting go' their young adult children.

Dermot's needs were rather different. His learning difficulties were more serious than Jason's, and were complicated by physical disabilities which made him unable to move around by himself. At the age of twenty-five he was still living with both parents. His specialist health care during his childhood was provided by a paediatric centre of excellence in another regional health authority. At the time of referral to the Community Mental Handicap Team, when Dermot was twenty-four, his parents were still taking him for his twice-yearly check-ups. The paediatrician had not known to whom to pass on his care! The keyworker appointed by the Community Mental Handicap Team was a physiotherapist who could accompany Dermot and his parents to his next check-up, and begin the process of phasing his care to local adult services. His mother's depression and back-ache pointed to the need for either more hands-on practical help at home or regular respite care or both. If preview had been operating these services could have been offered many years earlier with prevention in mind.

Jane was in her fifties, and was showing early signs of senility. She was losing some of her daily living skills, and her personal care had deteriorated. She was referred to the team for hospital admission because of complaints to the council housing department about the smell coming from her flat. Jane had become incontinent and was unable to manage a daily bath for herself or to do her extra laundry. She did not want to lose her home. An occupational therapist was able to work alongside the home help and district nursing services and help Jane acquire an acceptable level of cleanliness. Initially the home help organizer had felt Jane was not really eligible for this service, but her negative attitude and feelings of revulsion faded when she saw that other workers valued Jane enough to work closely with her.

The Community Mental Handicap Team works in the community and visits and assesses people in their own homes and places of employment and activity. It does not function from a remote out-patient clinic, and tries to be as accessible and useful a component of the network as it can. A great deal of the work of the Community Mental Handicap Team focuses on separation issues.

Learning from past mistakes

Will we learn from the mistakes of past generations? Will we understand the relationship between cause and effect? Will new human service systems be flexible enough to meet individual need, or merely be monuments to our own limited vision? Both the parent movement and more recently self-advocacy groups have stressed the importance of choice. Choice implies variety. Variety of opportunities in where to live, where to work and play and with whom. The institutional 'warehousing' model of care offered no choice of environment.

There are plenty of ideas to extend all manner of opportunity to people with learning difficulties living in community settings. For example, museums are becoming more accessible to people who want to touch an exhibit or interact with it. A national theatre project is being planned to introduce more people with mental handicap to the arts. A young woman with Down's syndrome recently gained the Duke of Edinburgh's Gold Award. Scout and Guide troops welcome children with disabilities as full members.

Optimism thrives on these examples of good practice. Sadly there is plenty of room for pessimism too. In order to build supporting services in the community, resources are being taken away from the shrinking hospital-based residential 'communities'. The quality of life there is not improving. Staff morale is invariably low and recruitment to mental handicap nursing is slow. Understandably new recruits to the nursing profession want to be part of the new developments in the community.

For those still living in institutional settings perhaps the happiest outcome would be for an alternative model, not a dumping ground.

Summary

Services for people with mental handicaps have followed successive historical trends and have grown up piecemeal. Today, services are at many different stages of a movement away from hospitals and towards care in the community, and their character and quality varies from one place to another. Children increasingly live with their parents or in foster homes, and have the choice of education in mainstream schools. Parent groups have won considerable advances in provision of services and are now fighting for full acceptance of their adult children in society. Carers can tap into a local network of special schemes which offer them extra help. In most parts of the country Community Mental Handicap Teams are starting to bring together professionals from different disciplines to discuss an individual's progress, to suggest strategies and to recommend expert help. In one area successive previews of potential need are planned to anticipate developmental crises and plan future care.

Notes

1. 1971 White Paper, *Better Services for the Mentally Handicapped.* HMSO.
2. G. Wyatt and C. Langmead, *Charnwood.* Lion 1987.
3. King's Fund Project paper, no. 24, *An Ordinary Life: Comprehensive Locally-based Residential Services for Mentally Handicapped People.* King's Fund Publishing Office, 14 Palace Court, London W2 4HT.
4. P. Jay, *Report of the Committee of Enquiry into Mental Handicap Nursing and Care.* HMSO, Cmnd 4768 − 1, 1979.
5. Ann Shearer, *Building Community with People with Mental Handicaps, their Families and Friends.* Campaign for People with Mental Handicaps and King Edward's Hospital Fund for London 1986.
6. *Who can Help? A − Z Directory of Services for Children and Adults with Disabilities in Wandsworth.* Wandsworth Social Services Department (Welbeck House, London SW18) 1986.
7. *London Directory of Services.* Royal Society for Mentally Handicapped Children and Adults, 123 Golden Lane, London EC1.
8. Edna Wallace, 'Preview' (*Social Work Today*, 1978).
9. Edna Wallace, 'Preview' (*APMH Newsletter*, 1987).
10. R. Blunden, *Individual Plans for Mentally Handicapped People*: a draft procedural guide, 1980. Mental Handicap in Wales, Applied Research Unit, Cardiff.

NINE

Imagining Possibilities

Three secrets are commonly kept from people with learning difficulties. The first is the secret of their handicap. There is a tendency to do things for him or for her, to make choices on their behalf, to decide what is good for them without putting corresponding energy into helping them come to terms with the reality of their situation. Among young adults the hardest thing for them to talk about is their anger and sadness about their handicap. Their habit is to use it as an excuse. The direction of their growth lies in expressing the sorrow and the anger, and in feeling understood and accepted. 'Sharing sad things' can be the beginning for people with mental handicaps in cultivating their strengths.

The second secret is the secret of mortality. Their parents will die. Good parents on whom they depend, who will fight for them and protect them and order life to suit their needs, these parents will die. Shielding handicapped people from the little losses, pretending they won't notice, does nothing to prevent the catastrophe of the final loss of their parents. Coming to terms with each small loss and each change, working through the anger and the grief towards genuine acceptance, striving for the maximum self-reliance and the widest network of relationships, this is the only way to prepare for the inevitable loss of parents by death. And this, too, is the only way in which all of us learn to face up to the inevitability of our own mortality.

The third secret is the secret of their sexuality. Others may have sexual partners, may marry and have children. For people with mental handicaps there is to be eternal childhood or masturbation filling the long, lonely hours. Sterilization or abortion are widely assumed necessary for a young woman, or if she has a child it will be taken away. Somehow the secret must be told, the nettle grasped. Sexual ignorance can be replaced by sexual education, unsocial behaviour exchanged for something more appropriate. With careful preparation satisfying relationships can often be achieved on the personal and sometimes also on the sexual level.

Pastoral care workers reading this book will have considered many opportunities of starting to reveal a little of these three secrets. Ideally the secrets will be told sensitively, gradually and when the occasion arises naturally. There is no question of going in flat-footed and brutally stripping away illusion, upsetting people with learning difficulties and their carers alike. It is rather by refusing to shut out all of the everyday chances: chances of working through grief at being different, chances of coming to terms with change and loss, chances of understanding and coping with the fact that people with mental handicaps are sexual people too. And pastoral care workers may also be able gently to challenge the collusion of parents or carers in the keeping of the three secrets, by gently showing them the daily opportunities of facing up to the realities.

A counselling approach

How is this gentle intervention to be achieved? Many times during this book the value of counselling has been stressed. Thus we make the claim that counselling is opportune when parents have heard that their expected baby may have mental handicaps and they are considering whether or not to have the pregnancy terminated. When parents hear news of their child's handicap, a type of bereavement counselling can help the task of mourning the perfect child who is lost and accepting the actual child who exists in reality. As each milestone for mainstream children is reached—milestones like starting school or leaving home or beginning work or choosing a boyfriend or girlfriend—counselling can help parents of a handicapped child to work through their sense of grief and loss and to mobilize their desire to develop their child's actual strengths. Counselling can lessen the need parents may have to deny that their handicapped child is a sexual person and so can enable them to start a suitable sexual education for him or her. Counselling can lessen the guilt which may prompt parents to cling unnecessarily to adult sons and daughters or to use handicap as a reason for preventing independence. What, then, is counselling, and what are pastoral workers to understand by a counselling approach?

The term 'counselling' is often loosely used in ways which differ from the sense used in this book. In the world of work the term 'career counselling' is sometimes used for interviews intended to reconcile an individual with lack of promotion or to discipline an employee for misdemeanours. In the field of handicap the term 'genetic counselling' is sometimes used to describe simply the giving of information about a genetic disorder, which may be coupled with a recommendation for avoidance or termination of pregnancy. The term 'counselling' is not used in this book to mean either asking questions, or imparting information, or giving advice, or influencing attitudes, or persuading towards a particular course of action, or manipulating a person for other ends.

Classic counselling comes from the practice of Carl Rogers[1] who by building a genuine relationship of trust with his clients made them feel accepted on their own terms and understood at a deep emotional level. Rogers found that his genuine understanding and acceptance enabled his clients to let go of their defences, to gain insight into their own behaviour and to realize that they could choose to behave differently. Rogerian counselling is characterized by being 'for' the client and by trusting the client's own potential for personal growth. These principles of Rogers are basic to later systems of counselling and to the counselling approach in general. If pastoral workers wish to adopt a counselling approach they can do no better than to start by improving their skills of careful listening and of responding with accurate empathy.

Carl Rogers set great store upon clients telling their own story in their own way and tended to intervene very little with interpretations, leaving the counselling hour relatively unstructured. Full Rogerian counselling therefore tended to take place over a considerable time, a matter of years rather than of months or weeks. It was strong on acceptance and insight (the *why* of change) but weaker on problem-solving skills (the *how* of change).

Now counsellors tend to intervene more actively and to

structure time more closely, making the whole process considerably shorter. They do this in various ways: by adopting the ideas and exercises of Fritz Perls and Gestalt therapy,[2] which focus always on the here and now: by using ideas from Eric Berne's school of Transactional Analysis,[3] which challenge compulsive rituals and which vividly show how past interactions between parents and child are influencing present choices and behaviour; by using guided fantasy in the manner of Jung and the school of Psychosynthesis. The Lifeskills movement[4] offers counsellors a whole battery of exercises and games which bring together the fruits of these various schools. Gerard Egan[5] has taught the skills of counselling, such as how to respond with empathy, how to confront constructively and how to help clients solve problems and set realistic goals. He has also analysed the counselling process itself, so that counsellor and client do not become stuck forever in the exploration of problems but move on to making decisions and planning the future.

Pastoral workers can see that counselling today is built upon the respect, empathy and genuineness originally inspired by Carl Rogers. But, whether carried out with individuals or with groups, it is often nowadays a lively and active art. Many workers who are not trained counsellors can borrow with advantage from the counselling approach and from counselling skills and methods.[6]

The 'wrong' choice

One of the first principles laid down by Carl Rogers was that counselling should be non-directive. So a counsellor working with parents who have heard that their expected baby will have a mental handicap will help those parents to make up their own minds whether or not to ask for a termination. The counsellor will encourage them to express their grief, anger, pain, fear and bewilderment; to tell each other their personal principles and how strongly or minimally they hold to them; to rehearse the facts as they understand them and to discover whatever else they need to know; to explore the probable outcome of either choice. The counsellor brings the parents as nearly as possible to the point where any decision they make will be an informed one. Counsellors may belong to a church which disapproves of such abortions or to a hospital department whose policy favours them. Personally, the counsellor may have strong convictions in one direction or another. What enables a counsellor to be non-directive is an overriding belief in the supremacy of conscience, in the moral autonomy of individuals, and in the rightness for those parents of a moral decision they have conscientiously taken. There can be pain for a counsellor if parents appear to make the 'wrong' choice; it is the pain of Christ who loved the rich young man but let him go (Mark 10.17—22). The man's freedom to accept or reject the choice before him was important enough for Christ to risk the pain.

Pastoral care workers as counsellors

It is clear that not everybody is suited to being a counsellor and not all pastoral workers will want to practise counselling skills and methods. Yet, for those who are prepared to listen with empathy, and are able to be non-judgemental and non-directive, the counselling approach has much to offer. It holds great potential for helping parents and carers of people with mental handicaps to understand themselves and their situation, to make informed and conscientious choices with regard to their charges and to plan realistically how to carry them out.[7]

The value of a counselling approach to people who themselves have mental handicaps is less clear. The classic 'talking treatment' has no place for those with little or no speech. Abstract reasoning will not succeed. Decisions which need the co-operation of parents and carers to carry them out cannot be reached in individual and confidential interviews with a handicapped person. Many choices are not appropriate for particular people, as is brought out in this account by Jenny Cooper:[8]

> Simon was an eighteen-year-old lad leaving hospital to live in the community. He was encouraged to make his own choices. He chose to spend some of his money on a tape-recorder. Some hospital staff felt he should only buy essentials, but we managed to convince them that he would

not go short of anything he needed. He loved music. It was a very important part of his life and this was a choice that most of us felt appropriate.

But he made another request which was not so easy to support. Simon wanted to stop going to the ATC. Was it wise to go along with such a decision? Simon's intellectual functioning was perhaps similar to a five- or six-year-old's. We would not let our five-year-old child decide not to go to school. Even if other activities could be organized for Simon to occupy his time, does he not need to learn that even adults have to do things they do not like doing?

Situations like Simon's lead some people to say that counselling methods are just not suitable for people with mental handicaps. And yet workers who succeed best with mentally handicapped people seem to have a lot in common with the best counsellors. They manage to convey respect, empathy and genuineness. They accept clients as they are. They communicate not intellectually but through the emotions and the senses. They maximize appropriate choice.

Counsellors have a repertoire of methods which suit people with mental handicaps very well: experiential learning, role-play, drama and mime, 'being' a chair or a garment or another person. Counsellors prize being concrete and specific, they value the honest expression of feelings and see this as a way to understanding reality and personal growth: people with mental handicaps are often geniuses of the concrete and the specific and the emotions because they cannot perforce express themselves otherwise. How can they gain the benefit of the counsellor's repertoire?

Whose job?

Pastoral care workers are busy people. Whether they are church people like clergy, parish workers or members of religious communities; whether they are health personnel like doctors, nurses, health visitors or ancillary workers; or whether they are members of different caring professions like social workers, counsellors, teachers, personnel officers or community workers: all are likely to have a common experience of staff shortages, cuts in resources and working under pressure. Many pastoral workers may feel that they have plenty to do without taking on responsibility for people with learning difficulties. Yet often this proves well within their competence.

A marriage counselling agency, whose counsellors already undertake relationships education with groups of parents, teachers and adolescents, was invited to run a course on relationships within a small residential home for adults with mental handicaps, and wondered how to respond. It was felt that such work was marginal to the agency's purpose and that the counsellors had no mental handicap training.

It was agreed that a counsellor from the agency should share the course with an outside professional who was used to working with people with severe learning difficulties. Together they devised and ran a successful course with staff and residents together. The course owed as much to the familiarity of the counsellor with relationships and sexuality as to the professional's expertise in method and resources.

It is likely that many pastoral care agencies could extend their scope to work with people with learning difficulties, without needing additional training. What is needed more is the interest and the will. In other cases pastoral workers can help people with mental handicaps by working with those who care for them more directly:

The same marriage counsellor was asked to run an in-service training day with teaching and care staff of a residential school for children with severe learning difficulties. The head teacher requested that the counsellor should lead staff in sharing the difficulties each member experienced from the sexual behaviour of pupils and in devising guidelines for the school's policy on education for sexuality and relationships. The counsellor's existing skills in experiential groupwork, combined with exercises adapted from the FPA handbook *Options for Change*, provided the main ingredients for a successful day.

Here the counsellor took care to discover what specialized resources were available but found the work with teachers and care staff of a special school very similar to the counselling agency's usual work with mainstream schoolteachers. Another example of indirect pastoral care for people with mental handicaps is afforded by this account of work with their parents:

A third experiment was a residential weekend with a group of Christian parents of adults with mental handicaps. The marriage counsellor's groupwork skills were valuable in leading discussions among the parents about their sons' and daughters' emergent sexuality, and about facing up to their own death and the prior education and provision they would like to arrange for these young adults.

The parents were high in their praise for this course, but many elements contributed to its success: the enthusiasm of the parent organizers, the expertise and access to relevant films and exercises of a specialist professional worker, the participation of young volunteers who ran a parallel course with the handicapped young adults, the generosity of the conference centre staff who gave the parents first-class meals and service, also the readiness to experiment of the chaplain, who produced some memorable and active liturgies. Any success resulted from careful joint planning and sharing of expertise, but the marriage counsellor's skills were used and appreciated, and the course would have been poorer without them.

It is probable that many pastoral care workers could involve themselves with other carers and with mentally handicapped people themselves as effectively as this counsellor. These were the general conclusions which the marriage counsellor came to after several similar ventures:

1. If you normally offer a pastoral service, do not conclude too hastily that you cannot offer it to people with mental handicaps, or to their parents, carers or teachers.

2. Do not pretend to an expertise that you do not have, but be prepared to share your skills with others who have a different expertise, who are perhaps already working with people with learning difficulties.

3. Expect initially to give a great deal of time to planning.

Try out your ideas first on those who work or live with the people concerned. Explain what you will try to achieve and ask whether the means you have in mind are likely to be suitable. Ask for other suggestions that are likely to work better.

4. Pick the brains of specialists in mental handicap for news of resources. Be prepared to adapt them to your own way of working and to the needs of the people you will work with. Review all the resources normally available to you to see which may be easily adapted for people with learning difficulties.

5. Before you start, make some effort to understand the life experience of people with mental handicaps, and of their parents, carers and teachers.

6. Consult your colleagues for ideas beforehand and share your experience with them afterwards. Do everything you can not to become isolated from your own agency and try to get them to own the work you are doing in their name.

The last point is crucial. The pastoral worker's ability to work effectively with people with learning disabilities, or with their parents, teachers and carers, is not the whole story. Political will is needed for pastoral care to reach these people. Existing agencies must be made to recognize that these are indeed 'their people'. Agencies need the will to seek extra staff and resources if they are to take on more work without neglecting their original purpose. If they cannot find the will, the alternative is to set up specialist services to ensure that proper pastoral care is given to those people with learning disabilities who are taking up their rightful places within the community.

Every specialist service is an admission of a certain failure, the failure of ourselves, of society, to include people with learning difficulties among us. Sometimes specialist services are needed as refuges, as stop-gaps, as catalysts, as centres of excellence. Always their main aim should be to do themselves out of a job, to encourage the mainstream services and the ordinary pastoral carers to take on their responsibilities towards people with learning difficulties.

Is normal life possible for everybody?

Pastoral workers who have persevered this far and found themselves broadly in agreement with this book's philosophy may yet ask themselves how realistic is this quest for a normal life. Most mentally handicapped people are only mildly so, as is evident from the percentages quoted in Chapter 1. Perhaps these can make progress towards an ordinary life within the community. But the others, what of them?

The word 'profound' means unfathomable, which is quite a good description of someone who is profoundly handicapped. It is so difficult to imagine what perception they can have of the world when they are unable to understand or use any form of language. Such a person will be totally dependent on someone else for food and drink, for warmth and shelter. He or she may have multiple impairments as well, such as deafness or blindness, or serious physical deformity. In addition he or she is likely to be doubly incontinent and may have severe epilepsy. When profound handicap seems to take an individual almost beyond the ordinary person's reach or understanding, what can we say then about progress towards a normal life?

Dr Jurgen Trogisch[9] describes two such profoundly handicapped children from his East German hospital, Daniel and Monika. He tries to imagine what Daniel and Monika might ask him if they could speak. These are some of the questions with summaries of his replies.

Daniel and Monika ask: 'Why can't we live as comfortably as other children do in our country?'

Dr Trogisch notes their institutional setting, with communal bath, shortage of personal cupboards, high window sills, and staff forever rushing about. He tries to face the contradiction between what we look upon as legitimate requirements for ourselves and the provision we concede to handicapped people.

Daniel and Monika ask: 'Why can't we be educated like all the other children in our country?'

Dr Trogisch asserts 'that all severely disabled people have some learning ability. However, it is important that they are taken along a small step at a time and that we do not allow what has been achieved to be lost. Frequently it is our lack of knowledge or lost sympathy with the patient, our failure to use our powers of observation and our unrealistic expectations' which hinder further learning.

Daniel and Monika ask: 'Why is it that you often don't understand what we want and what we are trying to tell you?'

Dr Trogisch marvels how, by careful observation and interpretation, sensitive parents and carers can understand and communicate. 'If you try to analyse this form of communication you find that it is very similar to the way a mother talks to her young baby.' We who have no disabilities have a real handicap when our embarrassment prevents us from engaging in this pre-verbal communication which uses face, voice, cadence, song, together with smell, taste, temperature and touch.

Daniel and Monika ask: 'Why are we so alone?'

Dr Trogisch is shocked by the lack of attention given to children in residential homes compared with the network of relationships at home between ordinary children and the adults who care for them. Many behavioural disorders stem simply from lack of personal attention and he advocates enlisting selected lay helpers and school pupils as personal friends.

Daniel and Monika ask: 'Why are our parents so unhappy?'

The answer is that their sense of grief and loss makes many parents feel helpless and they need pastoral carers to work through this loss with them and bring them to accept it. Only then can they help to create a sense of dignity in every area of their children's lives.

Daniel and Monika ask: 'What is the point of living at all, has our life any meaning?'

Dr Trogisch finds part of the answer in the experience of young adults tending them and people like them:

'It has made me question what is really important in life.'

'It has been an enriching experience, work has assumed a new meaning and purpose, I feel I am needed now.'

'I have become more serious minded and think more consciously about life.'

'I have become more tolerant, my own little problems don't seem so important any longer and I have learned to accept myself with all my own inadequacies. Above all, I have learned to appreciate the little pleasures in life, such as the sight of a table laid for a meal, and especially I thank God that he has shown me that love can achieve more than hate or force.'

Dr Trogisch concludes: 'Daniel and Monika have only very minimal abilities, some would say that they have none at all . . . But when I consider how both Daniel and Monika and other severely mentally disabled people have, by the very fact of their existence, brought about such changes in the lives of the young people I have referred to, I am tempted to suggest that they should be employed as teachers in our educational system because of the effect they could have.'

Dr Trogisch does not deny any of the difficulties entailed in caring for people with profound handicap; he recognizes that some people are afraid to meet children like Daniel and Monika and that deep shock and sadness can often be seen in the faces of friends and relatives who visit them. His account is challenging but it is not hopeless. It indicates what progress towards a more normal life might mean for Monika and for Daniel. It is in sharp contrast with the attitude which deems people with profound handicap as incapable of learning and merely requiring custody in a warehouse awaiting death.

Disorders of behaviour

Reluctance to accept people with mental handicaps into an ordinary community sometimes stems from the uneasy fear that they may behave violently or unpredictably. It is important to clarify that mental handicap does not of itself usually create disorders of behaviour, yet there are several reasons why people with mental handicaps do sometimes behave oddly. Lack of loving relationships or of meaningful activity will have repercussions on anyone's behaviour. Sometimes individual friends and people who will take a personal interest have to be sought deliberately on behalf of people with mental handicaps, perhaps from relatives or neighbours, from church or social groups, or as volunteers from among school children or unemployed or retired people. Programmes to extend their range of activities can be drawn up nowadays in consultation with all who have care of them and should be systematically followed.

The inability to articulate angry feelings can be highly frustrating and sometimes physical expressions of anger are the only means of expression available to an individual. Often the cause of the anger can be readily understood and steps can be taken to alter it.

One eight-year-old boy was very conscious of his elder sister's slowness. His bossy habit of making his sister play games his way led to complaints from him that she was pulling his hair. It was unhelpful to punish this teenage girl, but the situation was improved by addressing the rivalry between the siblings.

Psychiatrists and psychologists are trained to analyse what happens before and after aggressive outbursts, to consider clues to the cause of these patterns which repeat themselves again and again and to suggest remedies. They are also trained to recognize those unusual cases where the behaviour of children or adults is so unpredictable that it is dangerous for carers to be left alone with the individual. An apparent change in personality leading individuals to become very withdrawn or to injure themselves might signal depression. Losing skills, such as the ability to dress oneself or to remain clean and dry, could be due to depression which is treatable, or to a progressive organic brain syndrome, such as dementia. Yet, although such skilled assessment is sometimes necessary and should be readily accessible, pastoral workers can be assured that their own help in supporting healthy and fulfilling lifestyles for people with mental handicaps can go a long way towards preventing behavioural disorders from developing.

Outsiders or one of us?

This chapter started with three secrets which we, the clever people who can read books, conspire to keep from people with mental handicaps. But there is an even bigger secret which we contrive to keep from ourselves. This enormous

secret is that we are often quite stupid. From our childhood
we have been made ashamed of our stupidity and — our ears
ringing with 'Don't be silly!' and 'Have some common sense!'
and 'Don't be such a fool!' — we have striven to join the clever
ones. We know that this is the group which gets the fame and
the riches, the man or the girl.

Sometimes we doubt whether we will ever become truly
clever. It then suits us very well that there is a group who are
certainly more foolish than we are. Whether we call them
'mentally handicapped people' or 'people with learning
difficulties', that is where stupidity certainly resides. While
that group exists outside our own lives we do not have to
admit to our stupidity but, by the well-known defence of
projection, we can locate it among the outsiders. No wonder
it is difficult for us to support plans to bring the stupid ones
back into our community, for that would mean taking back
our projections and owning our own stupidity.

Yet there is a freedom in dropping the pretence of constant
cleverness and infallibility. There is a human camaraderie in
admitting our mistakes. It is a kindlier society where all of us
can let our weakness be seen and still be accepted.

Choosing where to walk

In St John's Gospel there is an account of Jesus talking to
Peter. Himself a free spirit who had walked the roads of
Judea and of his native Galilee, Jesus seems to have recognized
the same sense of freedom and self-reliance in his older friend
the fisherman.

> 'And further, I tell you this in very truth: when you were
> young you fastened your belt about you and walked where
> you chose; but when you are old you will stretch out your
> arms, and a stranger will bind you fast and carry you
> where you have no wish to go' (John 21.8 NEB).

For the person with a mental handicap, for Kevin, the
experience of walking where he chooses may never be his.
The task of pastoral care is to see that Kevin makes as many
of his own choices as possible and goes as far as ever he can.
It is for pastoral care workers to take up this book's assertion
that Kevin is indeed 'going somewhere'. Only so can we

realize that Kevin and we are all travelling together, and that we are the poorer for depriving ourselves of what Kevin has to give.

Notes

1. Carl Rogers, *Client-centered Therapy*. Houghton Mifflin (USA) 1981.
2. Gaie Houston, *Little Red Book of Gestalt*. Rochester Foundation 1984.
3. Thomas A. Harris, *I'm OK, you're OK*. Pan 1973.
   Eric Berne, *What Do You Say after You Say Hello?* Corgi 1975.
   Muriel James and Dorothy Jongeward, *Born to Win*. Addison-Wesley (USA) 1985.
4. Barry Hopson and Mike Scally, *Lifeskills Teaching Programmes*. Lifeskills Associates, Leeds, 1983.
5. Gerard Egan, *The Skilled Helper*. Brooks/Cole 1982.
6. Michael Jacobs, *Still Small Voice: an Introduction to Pastoral Counselling*. SPCK 1982.
   Michael Jacobs, *Swift to Hear: Facilitating Skills in Listening and Responding*. SPCK 1986.
7. Cliff C. Cunningham and Hilton Davis, 'Early Parent Counselling', chapter 15 in Craft, Bicknell and Hollins (ed.), *Mental Handicap*. Bailliere Tindall 1985.
   A. Cooklin and S. Hollins, 'Hugo Wasn't Invited', *Children and Handicap: a Dialogue about Family Intervention*. An Institute of Family Therapy training tape, 1987.
8. Jenny Cooper, 'Remember They Are Not Normal' (*Community Care*, 8 May 1986).
9. Dr Jurgen Trogisch, 'Congenital Subnormality: — the Rehabilitation of the Severely Mentally Handicapped', in *God and The Handicapped Child*. Christian Medical Fellowship 1982.

Useful Addresses

AFASIC—Association for all speech impaired children, 347 Central Markets, London EC1A 9NH (01 236 3632/6487)
Provides advisory service for parents including where to go for assessment. Actively works to increase speech therapy provision for language-disordered children and young people.

APMH—Association of Professions for Mentally Handicapped People, Greytree Lodge, Second Avenue, Greytree, Ross-on-Wye, Herefordshire HR9 7EG (0989 62630)
Promotes cooperation between parents and different professional groups.

Campaign for People with Mental Handicaps, 12A Maddox Street, London W1R 9PL (01 491 0728)
CMH campaigns for better services for all age groups of people with learning difficulties.

Church Action on Disability, Rev. John Peirce, Charisma Cottage, Drewsteignton, Exeter
An ecumenical campaign to encourage the participation of all disabled people in the worship, fellowship and ministry of the Church by increasing accessibility and changing attitudes.
Publishes a regular newsletter called *All People*.

Contact a Family, 16 Strutton Ground, London SW1P 2HP (01 222 2695)
CAF links families with a handicapped child through local self-help groups with the aim of offering support, friendship, practical help and information exchange.

CRUSE, Cruse House, 126 Sheen Road, Richmond, Surrey TW9 1UR (01 940 4818)
The national organization for widows, widowers and their children. Offers counselling, advice and guidance on practical

matters, opportunities for contact with other members and a range of publications.

DHSS
Direct dial number for free general advice and expert information on social security benefits: 0800 666555.

Down's Children's Association, 12-13 Clapham Common, Southside, London SW4 7AA (01 720 0008)
The DCA has an information and advice centre and a 24-hour helpline.

ESNS Consortium, Jack Tizard School, Finlay Street, London SW6 6HB
Develops resource materials for teachers working with children who have severe learning difficulties.

Family Planning Association, 27 Mortimer Street, London W1 (01 636 7866)
The Education Unit runs courses on personal relationships and sexuality for people working in the field of mental handicap.

Family Fund (formerly called The Rowntree Trust), PO Box 50, York YO1 1UY (0904 21115)
Offers financial support to parents of children under 16 who have severe handicaps. Individual applications are considered for the cost of washing machines, bedding, holidays and other expenses not covered by DHSS, Social Services or Health Services.

In Touch Trust, Mrs Ann Worthington, 10 Norman Road, Sale, Cheshire M33 3DF (061 962 4441)
Contact and information service for parents of children with mental handicap.

King Edward's Hospital Fund for London, Centre: 126 Albert Street, London NW1 7NF (01 267 6111), Publishing Office: 14 Palace Court, London W2 4HT (01 727 0581)
Involved in training, research and publications in health care management including mental handicap.

MENCAP (Royal Society for Mentally Handicapped Children and Adults), 123 Golden Lane, London EC1 (01 253 9433)
Provides a wide range of services for people with mental

handicap, their families and the professionals who work with them.

MAKATON Vocabulary Development Project, 31 Firwood Drive, Camberley, Surrey GU15 3QD (0276 61390)
The Makaton Vocabulary is a language programme which provides a basic means of communication using speech with signs and/or symbols, and encourages language development in people with mental handicaps (of all ages).

Richmond Fellowship, 8 Addison Road, London W14 (01 603 6373)
Residential therapeutic communities for young adults with mild learning difficulties. Also offer a part time course in pastoral care and counselling in London.

St Joseph's Centre, The Burroughs, Hendon, London NW4 4TY (01 203 3999)
A Pastoral Centre for people with mental handicap in the Westminster Diocese.

Strathcona Theatre Company, Strathcona Social Education Centre, Strathcona Road, Wembley, Middlesex (01 451 7419)
The members of the Company all have learning difficulties. Through its performances and workshops the Company works to change stereotyped views of mental handicap.

SPOD—Sexual and Personal Relationships of People with a Disability, 286 Camden Road, London N7 0BJ (01 607 8851/2)
Provides an advisory service to clients, families and counsellors.

ARC—The Association of Residential Communities for the Retarded. For details of member organizations contact ARC, PO Box 4, Lydney, Glos. GL15 6ST (0594 530398)
ARC is an affiliation of member communities providing a diverse range of high quality residential care for people of any age who have mental handicaps.

The Spastics Society, 16 Fitzroy Square, London W1P 5HQ (01 387 9571)
Provides many services for people with cerebral palsy including special schools, further education centres and residential care. Also offers advice and support, assessment,

holidays and courses, and publishes a newspaper, *Disability Now.*

Tuberous Sclerosis Association, Little Barnsley Farm, Milton Road, Gatshill, Bromsgrove, Worcs. B61 0N9 (0527 71898) A regular newsletter attempts to report all items of interest about T.S. The Association sponsors conferences and research.

Index